# *Whole Foods*
# KITCHEN · JOURNAL

*Karen*
*thank you for the*
*support, Bernie '89*

*Best Fishes Karen!!*
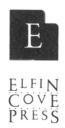

# B E R N I E   K U N T Z

ELFIN
COVE
PRESS

Published by: ELFIN COVE PRESS
P.O. Box 924
Redmond, Washington 98073-0924
USA

Copyright ©1989 by Bernie R. Kuntz
First printing 1989
Printed in the United States of America

**Library of Congress Cataloging in Publication Data**

Kuntz, Bernie, 1952-
   Whole foods kitchen journal / Bernie Kuntz.
   Includes index.
   1. Cookery (Natural foods)    I. Title
TX741.K86   1989
641.5'637—dc19          89-1591
                    CIP

ISBN 0-944958-36-2 soft cover

*Dedicated to my daughter*

*Nicole Jeaulé Mary*

# TABLE OF CONTENTS

# RECIPE LIST

## Chapter II
## VEGETABLES

Al's Horseradish Sauce
Another Spaghetti Sauce
Bob's Baked Potato
Boiled Asparagus
Broccoli with Sesame Seeds
Brussels Sprouts
Cheese Fondue for Two
Cilantro Lasagna
Cucumber Yogurt Sauce
Dried Tomato-Mushroom Quiche
Duffy's Baked Eggplant
Eggplant Tofu Casserole
Eggs and Mushrooms
Eggs with Zucchini
Fennel Dressing
French Dressing
Garlic Baked Tomatoes
Lucy's White Sauce
Mushroom Parsley Potatoes
Pizza Sauce
Sandy's Spinach-Mushroom Sauce
Sauce III Fast and Easy
Stuffed Mushrooms for Two
Sweet Potatoes
Tomatoes — Baked
Vegetable-Tofu Casserole and Spinach
   Noodles
Vegetarian Lasagna
Zucchini Spaghetti Sauce

## SALADS

4 Bean Salad
Beet and Bean Salad
Broccoli and Cauliflower Salad
Broccoli Sprout Salad
Cabbage-Garbanzo Beans-Carrot Salad
Carrot and Apricot Salad
Carrot Salad
Christine's Green Bean-Almond-
   Mushroom Salad

Fast and Easy Garbanzo Bean-Carrot Salad
Garbanzo Beans with Red Cabbage Salad
Garbanzo Beans with Basil
Garbanzo Beans-Tuna Salad in a Pita
Garden Salad
Jicama Salad
Potato Salad
Potato Salad with Dill and Tarragon
Potato Shrimp Salad
Raoul's Marinated Salad
Salami-Asparagus Salad
Spinach-Belgian Endive Salad
Spinach-Cauliflower Salad
Spinach-Chicken Salad
Spinach-Corn Salad
Spinach Salad with Cilantro
Spinach Toss Salad
Tabouly Salad
Tossed Green Salad
Tossed Green Salad with Bread Sticks
Vegetable-Pasta Salad with Anchovy
   Dressing
Vegetable Tuna Salad

## SOUPS

Acorn Squash Soup
Bean Soup
Borscht
Carrot Soup
Chicken Soup Mandy's Way
Clam Chowder I
Clam Chowder II
Cream of Brussels Sprouts and Mushroom
   Soup
Cream of Carrot and Mushroom Soup
Cream of Carrot Soup
Fish Chowder
Noodle Soup
Potato Soup
Rutabaga Turnip Soup
Sandy's Split Pea Soup
Tasty Turkey Soup

Thick Broccoli Soup
Yellow Split Pea Soup
Watercress Turkey Soup

**STIR-FRY**
Bok Choy and Broccoli Stir-Fry
Celeriac with Mixed Vegetables Stir-Fry
Snowpeas with Pinenuts Stir-Fry
Vegetable and Shrimp Stir-Fry

# Chapter III
## Seafood
Alaska Whitefish Stew
Almond Sole
Baked Cod
Baked Sea Perch
Barbecued Salmon
Barbecued Trout
Broiled Salmon Steaks
Broiled Salmon Steaks with Herbed
     Lemon Butter
Clam Linguini
Cold Lobster-Crab Pasta
Crab with Red Sauce
Easy and Quick Lunch Casserole
Easy Tuna Lunch Casserole
Fast and Delicious Salmon Tacos
Fresh Perch for Two
Frittata of Sorts
Geoduck Stew
Halibut Curry Salad
Halibut Patties
Halibut Sauté
Pasta Primavera with Salmon
Poached Salmon with Dill Sauce
Prawns
Ray's Teriyaki Fish Fry
Ronda's Fast Baked Halibut or Snapper
Roughy with Lime Juice
Salmon Quiche with Sun Dried Tomatoes
Sautéed Black Cod
Sautéed Prawns
Sautéed Squid with Mushrooms and
     Peppers
Seafood Banquet
Shrimp Quiche

Simple Black Cod
Snapper with Asparagus and Parmesan
     Cheese
Snapper with Mushrooms
Snapper with Mushrooms and Asparagus
Snow Crab Frittata
Snow Crab Paella
Steamed Salmon
Stuffed Salmon
Stuffed Trout
Uncle Bill's Barbecued Salmon or Trout
Uncle Bill's Steelhead on the Grill
Uncle Ray's Potato Fishcakes

# Chapter IV
## GRAINS/BEANS
7 Grain Cereal-Triticale Flakes-Bran
7 Grain Cereal and Triticale Flakes
AICR Cereal Mix
Amaranth Bread — No Eggs
Amaranth Seed-Brown Rice Flour Bread
     — No Eggs
Basic Quinoa
Basmati Rice with Tomatoes
Blueberry Muffins
Broccoli Tofu Bread — No Eggs
Brown Rice Pudding
Brown Rice Raisin Bread
Cheerio Date Granola
Chewy Granola-Dried Apple Muffins
Chocolate Chip Cookies
Cranberry Bread I
Cranberry Bread II
Flat Bread
Friday the 13th Granola
Kolache 86
Mary's Blueberry Muffins
Mixed Cereal
Mixed Rice
Molasses Granola
Nutmeg Rice
Oat-Barley Flakes Cereal
Oatmeal-Wheatena Cookies
Oats for Two
Orange Raisin Rice
Pie Crust

Quinoa and Amaranth Rye Bread — No
    Eggs
Pie Crust
Raisin Bread — No Eggs
Rolled Oats-Oat Bran Cereal
Saffron Rice
Scottish Oats
Toasted Quinoa
Whole Wheat Bread
Whole Wheat Blueberry Muffins

**PASTA**
Garlic-Oregano Pasta
Parsley Whole Wheat Pasta
Pasta Side Dish
Pasta Side Dish with Dried Tomatoes
Red Bell Pepper Pasta
Spinach-Whole Wheat Pasta
Whole Wheat and Bran Pasta

**BEANS**
All-Day Pot of Beans
Curried Lentils
Christine's Lone Star Caviar
Great Pot of Beans
Lentil Shrimp Salad
Lentil Turkey Salad
Lentils and Hocks

## Chapter V
## FRUIT
Apricot Jam with Sunflower Seeds
Apricot Papaya Jam
Baked Apples Deluxe
Banana Drink
Cantaloupe Drink
Fast Cheese Pie
French Style Apple Pie
Fresh Berry Pie
Fresh Fruit Salad
Fruit Dish for Two
Fruit Drink
Fruit Salad for Two
Fruit Salad with Strawberry Yogurt
Fruit Toss Salad
Papaya Jam with Almonds

Poppy Seed Fruit Salad (Bug Salad)
Prune Whip
Stuffed Strawberries
Yogurt French Bread

## Chapter VI
## POULTRY
Backed Chicken with Oyster Sauce
Baked Mustard Chicken with Garlic
    Carrots
Chicken Potato Pizza
Chicken Stir-Fry
Chicken Stir-Fry with Bifun Noodles
Chicken Strips
Chicken Verbier
Chicken with Grapes
Chin's Chicken Oriental
Cold Chicken Stir-Fry Salad
Curry Chicken
Fast Baked Chicken
Jeannie's Chicken and Steak Spray
Marinade for Chicken, Seafood, or Beef
Pancit
Quick Baked Chicken
Quick Chicken Enchiladas
Raoul's Chicken for Two
Roasted Chicken with Brussels Sprouts
Rolled Chicken Breast with Fettucine
Rosemary Chicken
Shiitake Marinated Chicken
Tamarind Chicken
Tarragon Game Hens
Turkey Breast with Spinach Stuffing

## Chapter VII
## MEATS
Asparagus-Spinach Meat Loaf
Broiled Lamb Steaks
Curried Lamb Steaks
Herb Spaghetti Sauce
Meatballs — High Fiber
Ray's Pepper Steak
Sautéed Venison
Sloppy Joes
Slow-Cooked Lamb Roast
Zucchini-Carrot Meat Loaf

## *DISCLAIMER*

This cookbook is designed to provide information and a variety of recipes. It is sold with the understanding that the publisher and author are not rendering medical advice.

Every effort has been made to make this cookbook as complete and accurate as possible. However, there may be mistakes both typographical and in content. Therefore, this cookbook should be used as a guide to healthy eating, not as an ultimate source on your diet decisions.

Always consult your physician before making major changes in your diet, especially if you have special dietary needs.

Publisher and author shall have neither liability nor responsibility for any problems caused or alleged to be caused directly or indirectly by information in this book.

**10**

# ACKNOWLEDGEMENTS

A giant thank-you to my family and friends for their moral support while writing this book, even through the delays. In particular, Mary Kresel, Dorothy Kuntz, Lucy Schumacher, Kate McConnon and Sandy Jirak for their help testing recipes and proofreading. And to those who contributed their original recipes to be included in this book, their names have been placed in the titles of their recipes so they can receive full credit.

Credit also to the American Institute for Cancer Research for allowing me to use their latest findings on important issues, such as cholesterol, salt, fiber and barbecuing. And the Alaska Seafood Institute, Evan Studio for their information on seafood, plus access to their artwork.

A special thanks to my friend, Ellen Serby, for invaluable information on how to write and publish a book and for setting me in the right direction.

— Bernie Kuntz


For more information on health, call the National Cancer Institute, 1-800-4-CANCER. Or write NCI, Office of Cancer Communications, Bldg. 31, Room 10A18, Bethesda, MD 20892.

Cover illustration by Ray Troll

Typesetting and Production by Grafisk Desktop Design
Edmonds, Washington
(206) 742-7015

# INTRODUCTION

It is proposed by all health organizations, such as the National Cancer Institute, the American Heart Association, the American Dietetic Association and the Academy of Science, that there is a strong connection between diet and heart disease, certain kinds of cancer, and obesity. While no "special" diet, food, or exercise will prevent disease, you can lower your risk by eating a diet with less cholesterol, less sugar and salt, less alcohol, fewer calories, and more complex carbohydrates and fiber.

*Whole Foods Kitchen Journal* is not just another lowfat cookbook. I have tried to make it into a journal for the health-conscious cook. Here is nutritional information which includes some of the latest findings from the American Institute for Cancer Research, the American Heart Association, and the American Dietetic Association on such topics as: Fat and Cholesterol, Fiber, Salt, and the importance of Vitamins and Minerals. Plus tips on healthy snacking, barbecuing, stir-frying, and choosing a lowfat cheese.

I have laid out this cookbook differently from the average cookbook. You will not find the chapters organized by course — soups, salads, main dishes, etc. Instead, the chapters are organized by types of food — vegetables, seafood, grains and beans, fruits, poultry, and meats. Along with 250 original, tested recipes to help you lower your cholesterol, salt, and sugar intake, and add fiber to your diet. While some meat recipes are included, I have deliberately kept the focus of this book on vegetables, seafood, grains and beans, fruits, and poultry. These recipes are easy and will not strand you in the kitchen for hours.

In each chapter, I try to provide enough information to acquaint you with whole foods and seafood, so they will be easy to start adding to your diet. I have listed more than 200 vegetables and fruits, both common and exotic, to choose from. There are a dozen grains listed, with their nutritional value and different available forms. A dozen types of beans are listed, with their nutritional value and cooking methods. To help you make the transition from eating meat daily to eating more seafood, I have provided nutritional information on different kinds of seafood, and a variety of recipes.

Some families can make the transition to a healthy diet very quickly. Most of us, though, find a gradual approach to be more effective. This is why a wide range of recipes is provided.

Think about it! Eating, day after day, year after year, adds up to the largest single influence on your body's well-being. We can increase the odds of living a long, healthy, energetic life. We make the choice every day. These changes do not have to be drastic. Start gradually by eating more fresh fruits and vegetables, grains, and beans. Substitute nonfat and lowfat dairy products for the whole fat ones. Start cutting back on meats, replacing them with seafood and poultry. Do not forget that a combination of diet and exercise is the most beneficial way to prevent disease and promote good health.

With the information and recipes provided in this cookbook, I hope *Whole Foods Kitchen Journal* truly works out to be *your* kitchen journal.

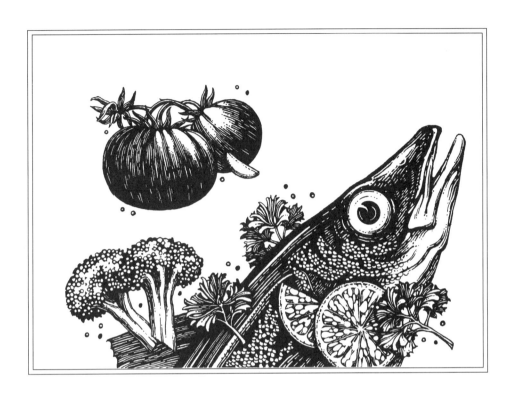

# NUTRITION

# AICR TARGET FOOD GUIDE

## SPARSE CONSUMPTION

Butter
Margarine
Lard
Mayonnaise
Whipped Cream
Cream
Oil
Chitterlings
Alcoholic Beverages
Deep-Fried Foods

Ice Cream
Non-Dairy Creamers
Non-Dairy Topping
Pastries
Sweet Rolls
Doughnuts
Cheese Puffs
Chocolate
Olives
Pecan Pie

Eclairs
Cheesecake
Custard Pie
Oil Salad Dressings
Fried Onion Rings
French Fries
Sour Cream
Cracklings

## VERY MODERATE CONSUMPTION

Fatty Beef
Salmon
Ham
Fatty Pork
Fatty Lamb
Cashew Nuts
Almonds
Chestnuts
Brazil Nuts
Goose Liver
Rainbow Trout
Coconut
Filberts
Goose
Herring

Tuna Canned in Oil
Fatty Veal
Peanuts
Peanut Butter
Pistachio Nuts
Sesame Seeds
Sunflower Seeds
Walnuts
Cream Cheese
Brick Cheese
Blue Cheese
Sausage
Parmesan Cheese
Pecans

Salami
Pepperoni
Charcoal-Broiled Meats
   and Fish
Whole Milk Yogurt
Whole Milk
Eggs
Frankfurters
Bacon
Swiss Cheese
Brie Cheese
Cheddar Cheese
Liverwurst
Bologna

## MODERATE CONSUMPTION

Skim Milk
1% Fat Milk
Part Skim Mozzarella
    Cheese
Tuna Canned in Water
Clams
Sole
Catfish
Bluefish
Bass
Oysters

Shrimp
Pike
Perch
Lobster
Cod
Flounder
Haddock
Scallops
Ricotta Cheese
Lowfat Yogurt
Baker's Cheese

Cottage Cheese
Sapsago Cheese
Fat Modified Cheese
2% Fat Milk
Buttermilk
Turkey
Lean Beef
Lean Lamb
Lean Pork
Lean Veal
Chicken

# WHAT'S LEFT?

## LIBERAL CONSUMPTION

Cantaloupe
Cucumber
Lettuce
Eggplant
Sprouts
Endive
Winter Squash
Sweet Potatoes
Spinach
Parsley
Chard
Carrots
Greens
Green Peppers
Celery
Corn
Beets

Cabbage
Cauliflower
Green Peas
Okra
Potatoes
Onions
Tofu
Bran Cereals
Pears
Peaches
Dried Beans and Peas
Fruit Juices
Grapefruit
Papaya
Oranges
Rhubarb

Watermelon
Raspberries
Whole Grain Pasta
Asparagus
Tomatoes
Cherries
Berries
Apples
Dates
Grapes
Pineapple
Plums
Brown Rice
Bananas
Escarole
Whole Grain Breads

*Source: American Institute for Cancer Research, Washington, D.C. 20069.*

# WHAT'S YOUR "R.Q."?
## (Refrigerator Quotient)

Do your eating habits reflect your knowledge and attitude about good nutrition? Your refrigerator may partly answer this question. The contents can tell something about your eating habits.

Here's a game to help you determine your R.Q. (Refrigerator Quotient) — one measure of how well your eating habits follow AICR's Dietary Guidelines to Lower Cancer Risk. All you need to play is the scorecard on page 23 and a pencil. Simply open your refrigerator (check your freezer, too) and count the number of foods you find in the various categories described below. Assign yourself points as instructed on the scorecard, and at the end add up these subscores to find your R.Q.

This scoring system is based on the fact that both visible fats and hidden fats in various foods need to be limited, and that eating a variety of fruits and vegetables helps to assure adequate intake of important vitamins, minerals, and dietary fiber.

This rating game is not intended to be a precise measure of the quality of your diet. It can, however, give you some *hint* as to how certain parts of your diet compare with the current guidelines.

### Part A: Fruits

Eating a variety of fruits regularly provides dietary fiber and a number of vitamins.

1. Count the different kinds of fruit and fruit juices in your refrigerator and freezer (and on your counters). For three (3) or more kinds, enter *1 point* in the blank for this section of the scorecard labeled (A-1).

2. Count any fruits or fruit juices that are high in vitamin C. Examples are cantaloupe, grapefruit, guava, oranges, papayas, and tangerines. For one or more of these, enter *1 point* in the blank labeled (A-2).

3. Count any fruit supplies that are high in beta-carotene. Examples are apricots (including canned or dried in your cupboards), cantaloupe, mangos, nectarines, papayas, persimmons, and watermelon. For one or more of these fruits, enter *1 point* in the blank labeled (A-3).

## Part B: Vegetables

Eating a variety of vegetables provides a balanced supply of vitamins and minerals.

1. Count the number of different kinds of vegetables and vegetable juices in your refrigerator and freezer. For three (3) or more kinds, enter *1 point* in the blank for this section of the scorecard labeled (B-1).

2. Count any vegetables or vegetable juices that are high in vitamin C. Examples are broccoli, collard or turnip greens, kale, hot chili or sweet bell peppers, watercress, and tomato juice. For one or more of these foods, enter *1 point* in the blank labeled (B-2).

3. Count any vegetable supplies that are high in beta-carotene. Examples are beet, collard, mustard and turnip greens; broccoli; carrots; chard; kale; mixed vegetables; pumpkin; spinach; sweet potatoes; watercress; winter squash; and carrot and tomato juices. For one or more of these vegetables, enter *1 point* in the blank labeled (B-3).

## Part C: Meat, Fish and Poultry

Reduction in fat consumption has been urged as a means of decreasing risk of cancer and heart disease. Meat products contain a significant amount of "hidden fat." They are an ideal place to start when looking to lower fat consumption.

1. Count the number of servings of low-fat foods that you have in your refrigerator and freezer. Examples are unmarbled, *lean* cuts of beef, pork, lamb, and veal, as well as chicken, turkey, most shellfish, frog legs, rabbit, squid, and venison. Enter the total in the blank on this section of the scorecard labeled (C-1).

2. Count the number of servings of high-fat meat and poultry

# R.Q. Scorecard

**Part A:**
**Fruits**

| (A-1) | + | (A-2) | + | (A-3) | = | Total Points Part A |

**Part B:**
**Vegetables**

| (B-1) | + | (B-2) | + | (B-3) | = | Total Points Part B |

**Part C: Meat,**
**Fish & Poultry**

| (C-1) | - | (C-2) | = | Result | | Total Points Part C |

If Result = 3 or greater, award 3 points for Part C.
If Result = 2, award 2 points for Part C.
If Result = 1 or 0, (same number of high-fat and lowfat), award 1 point.
If (C-2) is greater than (C-1), award 0 points.

**Part D: Dairy**
**Products**

| (D-1) | - | (D-2) | = | Result | | Total Points Part D |

If Result = 3 or greater, award 3 points for Part D.
If Result = 2, award 2 points for Part D.
If Result = 1 or 0, award 1 point.
If (D-2) is greater than (D-1), award 0 points.

**Part E: Rich**     Number
**Desserts**

Total Points Part E

If none, award 3 points for Part E.
If 1, award 1 point.
If more than 1, score 0 points for Part E.

**Total Score Parts A-E (R.Q.)**

23

products in your refrigerator and freezer. Examples are marbled or fatty red meats, duck and goose. Enter this number in the blank labeled (C-2).

## Part D: Dairy Products

This is another category of food in which the choices you make may have a significant impact on the amount of "hidden fat" that you are consuming.

1. Count the number of lowfat dairy products in your refrigerator. Examples are skim, 1% and 2% milk; buttermilk made from skim milk; chocolate *lowfat* milk; lowfat yogurt; lowfat cheese such as cottage, ricotta, sapsago, and farmer's; and part-skim mozzarella cheese, and all modified cheese labeled "lowfat." Enter the total number of these foods in the blank for this section of the scorecard labeled (D-1).

2. Count the number of high-fat dairy products in your refrigerator. Examples are whole milk, all types of cream, non-dairy creamers and toppings, eggnog, whole milk yogurt, and chocolate milk made from whole milk, and high-fat cheese such as blue, brick, brie, cheddar, colby, cream, edam, feta, gouda, whole milk mozzarella, muenster, provolone, and swiss. Enter the total number of these foods in the blank labeled (D-2).

## Part E: Rich Desserts

There is nothing wrong with rich foods from time to time, but when these foods are a *frequent* part of the diet, fat consumption is higher than the levels recommended to lower risk of cancer. It is also likely that there is little room left in the diet for a good supply of whole grains, fruits and vegetables. For these reasons, it is probably best to be very moderate in use of rich desserts.

Count the number of rich desserts in your refrigerator and freezer such as ice cream, pies, cheesecake, and frozen pastries. Enter the total number in the first blank in this section of the scorecard.

*Source: American Institute for Cancer Research, Washington, D.C. 20069*

## What Does Your R.Q. Tell You?

| Total R.Q. | Interpretation |
|---|---|
| 13-15 | EXCELLENT! Keep it up! |
| 10-12 | GOOD! Congratulations on your good eating habits! Are there a few small changes you'd be able to make that would bring your diet even closer to the guidelines? |
| 6-9 | FAIR. Some good habits, but still room for improvement. |
| 0-5 | NEEDS WORK. It's o.k. to eat high-fat food sometimes, but can you pick a spot to begin making some changes so that you get less fat and more nutrients? |

## What Doesn't Your R.Q. Tell You?

The important thing to keep in mind is that this game looks at only part of what you eat. It is the *total* diet that is important. When evaluating your results remember:

1. ***Portions Count.*** Large amounts of meats and cheeses *relatively* low in fat still add up to a lot of fat.
2. ***Added Fat Counts.*** Most people can use some added ("visible") fat such as margarine, oil and salad dressing each day and still keep total fat consumption within the 30% of calories goal, but amounts much beyond 2 Tablespoons per day should generally be avoided. Use of visible fats is not reflected in the R.Q. score.
3. ***Foods Eaten Outside the Home Count.*** If you eat out frequently, eating only lowfat foods at home but eating high-fat foods in restaurants can still make your fat consumption too high. Make careful choices outside your home, also.
4. ***Your Cupboards Count.*** A good diet is reflected in your cupboards, too. Use whole grains and legumes (dried beans and peas) frequently. Do snack foods high in fat and low in nutrients (such as cookies, chips, etc.) fill up your cupboards? Checking your cupboards might prove enlightening.

# FAT AND CHOLESTEROL

Fat provides energy, helps form cell membranes, promotes production of certain hormones, absorbs the fat-soluble vitamins A, D, E, and K, promotes proper growth, and helps regulate body temperature. Experts agree that some dietary fat is vital to good nutrition. But experts also agree there is strong evidence that excessive fat in the diet can contribute to disease. Heart disease, cancers of the colon, breast, and endometrium, and, of course, obesity are all correlated with a high-fat diet.

For most Americans, fat supplies more than 40 percent of their total calories, and 16 percent of these fat calories are from animal sources (saturated fat). By comparison, only 16 percent of total calories in the traditional Japanese diet are derived from fat, and most of this fat comes from vegetable sources (polyunsaturated fat). This high saturated fat intake of Americans seems to affect our rate of breast cancer, which is 85 percent higher than that of Japan. The American Institute of Cancer Research recommends reducing fat intake to 30 percent or less of total calories, and aiming to lower the average 16 percent of saturated fats to 5 percent. Cholesterol intake varies with individual needs such as body size, energy, and nutritional needs. The American Heart Association guidelines recommend cholesterol intake of less than 100 milligrams per 1000 calories and not to exceed 300 milligrams per day.

**There are three groups of fat:**

*1. Saturated fat* — Usually a "hard" fat, solid at room temperature. Saturated fats are found in animal sources such as red meat, poultry, whole milk dairy products, and lard. Saturated fats can also be found in certain types of "tropical" oils, notably coconut and palm oils. These oils contain between 51-92 percent saturated fats.

*2. Polyunsaturated fat* — Usually liquid, soft even when refrigerated. Polyunsaturated fats, found in fish and vegetable sources, contain linoleic acid, an essential fatty acid for proper digestion.

26

Good polyunsaturated choices are:
- Safflower oil ............74% polyunsaturated
- Sunflower oil ...........64% polyunsaturated
- Corn oil ...............58% polyunsaturated
- Soybean oil. ............57% polyunsaturated

*3. Monounsaturated fat* — Cancer researchers give this fat higher health marks than polyunsaturates, and it is generally not considered harmful to your heart. Monounsaturates are found in olive, avocado, and rice oils.

Because medical authorities have been telling us to cut down on our intake of saturated fats, in the past decade many of us have shifted to polyunsaturated fats. But now, to confuse us even more, there appear to be "good fat," "bad fat," and fats that are both "good and bad." **Saturated fat** increases low-density lipoproteins (or bad cholesterol) in our blood stream. Some researchers consider this a major contributor to cardiovascular disease. **Polyunsaturated fat**, while reducing levels of LDL's (bad cholesterol) in the blood, may also reduce the high-density lipoproteins (good cholesterol) needed for good health. **Monounsaturated fat** may wash out LDL's (bad cholesterol) while leaving a healthy level of HDL's (good cholesterol). New research suggests monounsaturated fat may actually reduce risk of cardiovascular disease.

---

### *What Does Your LDL (bad cholesterol) Count Mean?*

**LDL milligrams/deciliter**

Below 100 — "Ideal" level entailing very low risk.
100-120 — Low risk, eat healthy to keep it that way.
120-175 — Moderate risk, definite indication to lower cholesterol through diet modification.
Above 175 — HIGH risk. If diet alone doesn't lower cholesterol, drugs may have to be used.

Note: 200 mg/dl is average for many middle-aged Americans.

---

Last but not least is a new look at fish. It is believed by the American Institute of Cancer Research and other experts that fish oil, with its high-quality polyunsaturated oil known as omega 3 fatty acid, may alleviate high blood pressure and reduce chances of heart and blood vessel diseases; it may play an important role in protection against breast and prostate cancers; and may also help inflammation in cases of arthritis and asthma.

Omega 3 fatty acids are polyunsaturated like fatty acids in most vegetable oils, but they are structurally different and believed to influence a number of diseases. Research indicates that consumption of fish oils can help reduce levels of triglycerides and cholesterol, while raising the HDL (good cholesterol) levels, all beneficial in the prevention and treatment of heart disease. It is premature to state that fish oil has been proven effective in prevention and treatment of disease. Experts are excited about studies indicating that eating fish just three times a week may reduce your risk of heart disease. However, the use of fish oil supplements is unwise and not recommended.

The American Institute of Cancer Research and many other medical authorities emphasize that these and other recent findings on fat are subject to change as research continues around the world. Whatever their differences, experts are all telling us to CUT DOWN ON FATS OF ALL KINDS. Consumers should aim for an even balance in their diets including saturated, polyunsaturated, and monounsaturated. The American Heart Association's new health guidelines advise consuming no more than 30 percent of total daily calories in the form of fat. The Cancer Research Institute aims lower, recommending no more than 20-25 percent of total daily calories in the form of fat. The national average is 40 percent.

A strict menu or drastic sacrifices are not needed; just gradual modifications will help you lower your fat intake.

**How to Calculate Fat**
If you know the number
of grams of fat, you can
derive the numbers of calories.
Simply multiply the fat grams times 9.
1 fat gram = 9 calories

**How to lower fat intake:**

- Use fish or skinless poultry more often than red meat.
- Trim all excess fat off before cooking and use a cooking method that helps eliminate fat, such as roasting, grilling, baking, steaming, or broiling, instead of frying foods in fat.
- Use skim, nonfat, or lowfat dairy products. If this is hard for you, start out mixing $1/2$ whole milk and $1/2$ nonfat until you like the change. Cut sour cream with yogurt; serve ice milk instead of ice cream.
- Choose lowfat foods when you shop, such as grains, beans, fish, fresh vegetables, and fruits.
- Substitute broth for oil or margarine in cooking.
- Read labels to determine amounts and type of fat in packaged foods. Consider what you put into your body.
- Limit your intake of fats and oils that you add to foods in cooking and at the table, particularly those high in saturated fat, such as butter, lard, cream, heavily hydrogenated fats (some margarines), shortenings, and foods containing coconut or palm oil.

## Substitute the following lowfat foods for high-fat ones:

| HIGH-FAT FOOD | LOWFAT FOOD |
|---|---|
| Whole milk | Skim milk<br>Buttermilk<br>Nonfat powdered milk |
| Bacon | Chicken (or Canadian bacon) |
| Bologna, frankfurter, sausage | Chicken or turkey<br>Lean, thinly sliced beef |
| Avocado | Cucumber<br>Zucchini<br>Lettuce |
| Creamy or high-fat cheeses | Lowfat cheese<br>Cottage cheese |
| Ice cream | Ice milk<br>Frozen lowfat yogurt |
| Nuts | Fruit or vegetable snack |
| Hot fudge sundae | Frozen yogurt or ice milk with sliced or crushed fruit |
| Ground beef | Extra lean or lean beef with all fat trimmed |
| Fatty pork (spare ribs, ground pork) | Well-trimmed lean pork (leg, ham) |
| Sour cream | Lowfat yogurt<br>Imitation sour cream |
| Regular salad dressing | Reduced calorie salad dressing<br>Vinegar<br>Lemon juice |
| Cream | Skim milk |
| Fried egg | Poached or baked eggs |
| Liver | Lean meat<br>Chicken<br>Fish<br>Veal<br>Lowfat cheese |

| HIGH-FAT FOOD | LOWFAT FOOD |
|---|---|
| Hot dogs and hamburgers on a cookout | **Chicken** <br> **Skewered shrimp** <br> **Broiled fish** |
| Peanut butter and jelly sandwich | **Turkey breast** <br> **Chicken** <br> **Water-packed tuna** <br> **Crabmeat or shrimp salad** <br> **Lowfat cheese** |
| Stopping at a fast food restaurant on a long car trip | **Pack a homemade meal of lean broiled chicken, fruits, and raw vegetables** |
| Cream pie | **Unfrosted cake, made with less fat than the recipe calls for** |
| Potato chips | **Raw vegetables** <br> **Whole grain crackers** <br> **Pretzels** |
| Sardines | **Shrimp** <br> **Lobster** |
| Breakfast sausage | **Toast with cottage cheese** |
| Whipped cream | **Whipped evaporated skim milk (the bowl and beaters must be thoroughly chilled)** |
| Oil or mayonnaise dressing on a cold pasta salad | **Tomato sauce** <br> **Yogurt laced with herbs** |
| Chocolate | **Candy (if you must have it) that contains no chocolate** <br> **Sweet wafers made with no fat** |
| Hot chocolate or chocolate milk (made with whole milk) | **Hot chocolate or chocolate milk made with skim or lowfat milk** <br> **Strawberry or raspberry syrup mixed into skim or lowfat milk** <br> **Hot or cold lemonade** <br> **Fruit juice** <br> **Skim milk "blenderized" with raw fruit such as bananas or strawberries** |

*Source: American Institute of Cancer Research, Fall 1987 Newsletter, Issue 17*

## KEY WORDS

To understand fat-controlled and low-cholesterol diets these definitions are helpful:

**Atherosclerosis** is a disease in which fatty deposits collect on the inside of the artery wall. These deposits add up over many years, narrowing the channel through which blood flows. Atherosclerosis increases the risk of heart attack and stroke.

**Cholesterol** is a waxy material used in many of the body's chemical processes. Everyone needs cholesterol for good health, but too much cholesterol in the blood is associated with development of premature coronary heart disease and atherosclerosis. Cholesterol is found only in foods of an animal origin and is also manufactured in the blood. The American Heart Association recommends reducing the daily intake to no more than 300 milligrams of cholesterol from dietary sources.

**Triglycerides** are fats that are carried in the blood and are stored in the body as body fat. Triglycerides are made by your body from foods which you have eaten. Too many blood triglycerides may damage the blood vessels and increase your chance of developing coronary heart disease.

# FIBER'S ROLE IN GOOD HEALTH

Fiber is an important food element, and most plant foods contain many fibers. Foods high in fiber tend to be low in fat and simple sugars. These fibers, especially the polysaccharide ones, are important in the human diet. Other fibers are cellulose, pectin, hemicellulose, lignins, gums, and mucilages. Dietary fiber — those found in foods and not digested by the body — are of particular interest. Recent research has linked fiber to preventive benefits with respect to the following:

- **Weight control.** A diet high in fibrous foods promotes satiety and can promote weight loss, if those foods displace concentrated fats and sweets.
- **Constipation and diarrhea.** Some fibers attract water into the digestive tract, thus softening the stools. Some form gels, helping to solidify watery stools. By the one mechanism, they help relieve constipation, and by the other, they help relieve diarrhea.
- **Hemorrhoids.** Softer stools ease elimination for the rectal muscles and reduce the pressure in the lower bowel, creating less likelihood that rectal veins will swell.
- **Appendicitis.** Fiber helps prevent compaction of the intestinal contents, which could obstruct the appendix and permit bacteria to invade and infect it.
- **Diverticulosis.** Fiber exercises the muscles of the digestive tract so that they retain their health and tone and resist bulging out into the pouches characteristic of diverticulosis.
- **Colon cancer.** Some fibers speed up the passage of food materials through the digestive tract, thus shortening the "transit time" and helping to prevent exposure of the tissue to cancer-causing agents in food. Some fibers bind bile (described in Chapter 4) and carry it out of the body; this is also thought to reduce cancer risk.
- **Blood lipids and cardiovascular disease.** Fiber binds lipids such

as bile and cholesterol and carries them out of the body with the feces so that the blood lipid concentrations are lowered, and possibly the risk of heart and artery disease as a consequence.

- **Blood glucose and insulin modulation.** Monosaccharides absorbed from some complex carbohydrates, in the presence of fiber, produce a moderate insulin response and a more even rise in blood glucose. Insulin levels are high in obesity, cardiovascular disease, and diabetes (Type II), so this effect of fiber may be beneficial in terms of all three diseases.
- **Diabetes control.** Thanks to its effects on blood glucose, fiber helps to manage diabetes. Persons with mild cases of diabetes, given high-fiber diets, have been able to reduce their insulin doses.

It makes sense to increase the fiber in our diet, if only to keep our bowel action regular. Most high-fiber foods are delicious, satisfying, low in fats, and are not loaded with excess calories — four large advantages in a country where obesity, cancer, and heart disease are major health problems.

## *HOW MUCH IS TOO MUCH?*

The question of whether *excessive* fiber might be harmful, and what the ideal intake may be, remains to be answered. One concern about fiber is that both forms, soluble and insoluble, can block mineral absorption. Many researchers believe that such nutrient losses due to fiber would be insignificant in well-nourished individuals, and that after several months on a high-fiber diet, the body adapts and extracts the minerals from foods more efficiently. People who have marginal or inadequate intakes of vitamins and minerals — including the elderly, those on low-calorie diets, and children — may be likely to develop nutrient deficiencies on high-fiber diets. Clearly, fiber is like all other nutrients in that "more" is only better up to a point. Too much is no better for you than too little. Purified fiber is not as beneficial as fibers of food; purified fiber is empty of nutrients, while food fiber is loaded with them.

# SOME HIGH FIBER FOODS

|  | Grams of Fiber |
|---|---|

**Raw Fruits:**
Apple, 1 medium . . . . . . . . . . . . . . . .3.5
Avocado, 1 medium (16 oz.) . . . . . . .4.7
Banana, 1 medium . . . . . . . . . . . . .2.4
Blackberries, 1 cup . . . . . . . . . . . . .5.9
Blueberries, 1 cup . . . . . . . . . . . . . .4.0
Cantaloupe, 1/4 melon . . . . . . . . . . .1.0
Dates, 1 cup pitted . . . . . . . . . . . . .4.1
Dried prunes, 3 . . . . . . . . . . . . . . . .3.0
Guava, 1 medium . . . . . . . . . . . . . .5.6
Loganberries, 1 cup . . . . . . . . . . . .4.3
Mango, 1 medium . . . . . . . . . . . . . .1.8
Orange, 1 medium . . . . . . . . . . . . . .2.6
Papaya, 1 medium . . . . . . . . . . . . . .2.7
Peach, 1 medium . . . . . . . . . . . . . . .1.3
Pear, 1 small . . . . . . . . . . . . . . . . . .2.5
Persimmon, 1 medium . . . . . . . . . . .2.7
Raspberries, 1 cup . . . . . . . . . . . . . .6.8
Strawberries, 1 cup . . . . . . . . . . . . .3.0

**Cooked Legumes:**
Baked beans, 1/2 cup . . . . . . . . . . . .11.0
Kidney beans, 1/2 cup . . . . . . . . . . .7.3
Lima beans, 1/2 cup . . . . . . . . . . . . .4.5
Navy beans, 1/2 cup . . . . . . . . . . . . .6.0

**Cooked Vegetables:**
Broccoli, 1/2 cup . . . . . . . . . . . . . . . .2.2
Brussels sprouts, 1/2 cup . . . . . . . . . .2.3

|  | Grams of Fiber |
|---|---|

Cabbage, white or red, 1/2 cup . . . . . . .1.4
Carrots, 1/2 cup . . . . . . . . . . . . . . . . .2.3
Carrots, 1 raw . . . . . . . . . . . . . . . . .3.0
Corn, 1/2 cup . . . . . . . . . . . . . . . . . .2.9
Green peas, 1/2 cup . . . . . . . . . . . . .3.6
Green pepper, raw, medium . . . . . . .2.4
Parsnips, 1/2 cup . . . . . . . . . . . . . . .2.7
Potato, 1 medium . . . . . . . . . . . . . .3.8
Spinach, 1/2 cup . . . . . . . . . . . . . . . .3.2
Turnips, 1/2 cup . . . . . . . . . . . . . . . .3.2

**Grains:**
Barley, 1/4 c. = 1 cup cooked . . . . . . . .3.5
Brown rice, 1 cup cooked . . . . . . . . . .1.7
Buckwheat, 1/3 c. = 1 cup cooked . . . .6.4
Millet, 1/4 c. = 1 cup cooked . . . . . . . .1.9
Oats, 1 cup cooked . . . . . . . . . . . . . .0.5
Popped corn, 1 cup . . . . . . . . . . . . .2.5
Rye berries, 1/4 c. = 1 cup cooked . . . .1.4
Rye bread, 2 slices . . . . . . . . . . . . . .5.4
Rye wafers, 3 . . . . . . . . . . . . . . . . . .2.3
Wheat bran, crude — 1 cup . . . . . . . .4.7
   1 Tablespoon . . . . . . . . . . . . . . . .0.3
Wheat bread, 1 slice . . . . . . . . . . . . .1.4
Wheat bulgur, 3/4 c. = 1 cup cooked . .2.2
Wheat germ, 1 cup . . . . . . . . . . . . . .2.0
   1 Tablespoon . . . . . . . . . . . . . . . .0.3
Wheat spaghetti, 1 cup . . . . . . . . . . .3.9

Over the past 50 years the consumption of fresh fruits and vegetables has dropped significantly, while consumption of processed fruits and vegetables (with 25% of the fiber removed) has almost doubled. The average American diet offers only 6-10 grams of fiber a day. While no recommended daily allowance has been set for dietary fiber, a reasonable target to shoot for would be 20-25 grams per day. Shop for whole foods, fresh vegetables, fruits, unrefined grains, and legumes. A diet of whole foods can provide 25 grams of fiber per day.

Sources:
    1. *Understanding Nutrition 4E,* by Whitney and Hamilton, 1987, pages 71-74, Table 3-3, page 73.
    2. *National Cancer Institute Publication No. 87-2878, December 1986, page 4. "Dietary Fiber and Disease,"* by D.P. Burkett, ARP Walker, and N.S. Painter, in the *American Journal of Medical Assoc. 299:-1068-1074, 1974.*
    3. *The Complete Eater's Digest & Nutrition Scoreboard,* by Michael F. Jacobson, Ph.D., 1985, pages 38-39.
    4. *National Cancer Institute Publication No. 87-2878, December 1986, pages 8-9.*

# *SHAKE THE SALT HABIT!*

You can reduce salt without reducing flavor. The average American consumes 4,000-8,000 milligrams of salt each day. It is estimated that we need about 230 milligrams of sodium each day (approximately $1/10$ of a teaspoon of salt). The American Heart Association suggests lowering sodium intake to 2,000 milligrams each day to reduce the risks of HYPERTENSION, HIGH BLOOD PRESSURE, and HEART DISEASE.

Some of the sodium-filled additives are listed on page 37. The only way to avoid all these additives is to avoid processed foods.

Low-sodium shopping and cooking does not have to be boring or flavorless. There are ways to reduce the amounts of salt in our diets and still enjoy flavorful foods.

**1. Read Labels**
Reading labels is very important when reducing salt intake. It is

believed that 30% of the average American adult consumption of salt originates in the processed foods we buy. Read labels and start choosing low-salt or no-salt products.

## 2. Start Eliminating the "Extra" Salt Used at the Table

Use less and less until the salt shaker is gone from the table altogether ($^1/_4$ of your salt intake is found here). To introduce change in the "salt habit," start by slowly eliminating its use in cooking. Adding salt to the water in which you cook rice, pasta, or vegetables is NOT necessary, especially when pasta and rice are often served with sauces.

## 3. Think About Doing More Cooking from Scratch

Leave the salt out, or at least cut it back. Season foods with fresh lemon or lime juice, fresh garlic, onions, salt-free onion and garlic powders, spices, and herbs. These are all great flavors and you will never miss the salt.

*Sources:*

  *1. Shaking the Salt Habit, American Heart Association*

  *2. Food Marketing Institute, Washington, D.C. Sodium Sense, developed in cooperation with Food and Drug Administration and National High Blood Pressure Education Program.*

  *3. The Complete Eater's Digest and Nutritional Scoreboard, by Michael F. Jacobson, Ph.D., pages 73-86.*

  *4. Coop Food Facts by Evelyn Roehl*

### GAMASIO (Sesame salt)

Mix 10 parts roasted sesame seeds with 1 part salt. Grind or mash together.

### HEART ASSOCIATION HERB MIX

$1/2$ teaspoon cayenne pepper
1 Tablespoon garlic powder
1 teaspoon each: basil, thyme, parsley, savory, mace, onion powder, black pepper, sage

### LINDA'S SEASONING SALT—NO MSG        Approximately $3/4$ cup

$1/2$ cup lite salt
3 teaspoons paprika
$1/4$ teaspoon celery seed
$1/2$ teaspoon garlic powder

Combine all ingredients and use in place of salt.

# VITAMINS AND MINERALS

Vitamins are among the most essential nutrients in our diets. Yet knowing just the "ABCs" of vitamins does not give a complete picture of vitamin benefits. It's important to understand how vitamins interact with other vitamins, with minerals, and with non-nutritive compounds, to do their vital work in maintaining good health.

In some cases, vitamins influence the absorption or utilization of other nutrients and elements, and in other cases they help the body protect itself against toxic compounds. Here are some of the ways vitamins and minerals help and protect the body.

## Interactions That Help
- Adequate vitamin E improves the body's use of vitamin A.
- Vitamin C enhances the absorption of iron when both are consumed at the same meal.
- Vitamin B2 is needed for the body's proper use of vitamin B6.
- Niacin, vitamin B2 (riboflavin) and vitamin B6 are all needed to prevent pellagra, a disease formerly linked only to niacin deficiency.
- Vitamin D regulates levels of calcium and phosphorus in plasma, a function necessary for bone mineralization.
- Vitamin D also regulates the absorption of calcium in the intestines.
- Vitamin E reduces some, but not all, signs of zinc deficiency, leading researchers to believe that the two nutrients have somewhat similar roles in strengthening red blood cells against the stress of oxidation.
- Zinc affects the body's need for and use of folate.
- Vitamin E and selenium act together as antioxidants in cells.
- Vitamin A deficiency is associated with changes in iron metabolism and resulting anemia.

## Interactions That Protect
- Vitamin E protects against harmful effects of silver, mercury, and lead.
- Selenium reduces the toxicity of mercury, silver, and cadmium.
- Vitamins E and C inhibit formation of the potent carcinogen nitrosamine from nitrates found in foods, smoke, and many other sources.

*Source:s:*
*1. "Vitamin Interactions," by The Vitamin Nutrition Information Service of Hoffman-LaRoche Inc., May 1985.*
*2. American Institute for Cancer Research Newsletter, 1987.*

## VITAMINS

| | BEST SOURCE | FUNCTION | DEFICIENCY SYMPTOMS |
|---|---|---|---|
| Vitamin A | Yellow fruits and vegetables, apricots, cantaloupe, squashes, watermelon, carrots, peas, kale, collards (green leafy vegetables), carrot juice, milk products, fish liver oil, liver. | Growth and repair of body tissues, bone and tooth formation, visual purple production (necessary for night vision). | Night blindness, loss of smell, fatigue, tooth decay (impaired formation of tooth enamel). |
| Vitamin B1 Thiamine | Wheat germ yeast, whole grains, nuts, fish, poultry, beans. | Carbohydrate metabolism, appetite maintenance, nerve function, growth and muscle tone. | Heart irregularity, nerve disorders, fatigue, loss of appetite, forgetfulness. |
| Vitamin B2 Riboflavin | Whole grains, green leafy vegetables, yogurt (lowfat), brewer's yeast, asparagus. | Necessary for fat, protein, and carbohydrate metabolism. Cell respiration, formation of antibodies and red blood cells. | Eye problems, cracks in corner of mouth, digestive disturbances. Severe deficiency is rare in the U.S. |
| Vitamin B3 Niacin | Tuna, salmon, chicken (light meat contains 50% more B3 than dark meat), milk products, brewer's yeast, peanuts, peanut butter. | Helps living cells generate energy. Fat, carbohydrate, and protein metabolism. Health of skin, and blood circulation. | Fatigue, irritability, loss of appetite, skin disorders, depression, diarrhea (pellagra). |
| Vitamin B6 Pyridoxine | Fish, poultry, lean meats. | Metabolism, formation of antibodies, maintains sodium and potassium levels (nerves). | Nervousness, dermatitis, blood disorders, muscular weakness, insulin sensitivity, anemia. |

| | BEST SOURCE | FUNCTION | DEFICIENCY SYMPTOMS |
|---|---|---|---|
| Vitamin B12 | Eggs, cheese, milk, fish. | Metabolism, maintains healthy nervous system, and blood cell formation. | Pernicious anemia, nervousness, fatigue, brain degeneration. |
| Vitamin C | Red or green bell peppers, the cabbage family, most vegetables (like broccoli, Brussels sprouts, rutabagas). Citrus fruits, rosehips, and sprouts. | Helps heal wounds, strengthens blood vessels, collagen maintenance, and resistance to infection. | Bleeding gums, slow healing wounds, poor digestion, aching joints, nosebleeds, bruising. |
| Vitamin D | Fortified milk, milk products, eggs, fish, fish oil. | Calcium and phosphorus metabolism (bone formation), heart action, nervous system maintenance. | Poor bone growth, rickets, nervous system irritability. |
| Vitamin E | Vegetable oils, green vegetables, wheat germ, eggs, sweet potatoes. | Protects red blood cells, inhibits coagulation of blood, protects fat soluble vitamins. | Muscular wasting, gastrointestinal disease, heart disease, abnormal fat deposits in muscles. |

Source: AICR, Complete Eater's Digest and Nutrition Scoreboard by Michael F. Jacobson, Ph.D. Nutrition Almanac, John Kirschman, director

## MINERALS

| | BEST SOURCE | FUNCTION | DEFICIENCY SYMPTOMS |
|---|---|---|---|
| Calcium | Milk products, green leafy vegetables, shellfish, tofu. | Strong bones, teeth, tissue, and muscles. Regulates heart action, nerve function and blood clotting. | Soft brittle bones, leg and back pain, heart palpitations, osteoporosis, loss of bone tissue. |
| Iron | Poultry, fish, eggs, leafy vegetables, beans (navy, black, and soybeans). | Hemoglobin formation, improves blood quality, increases resistance to stress and disease. | Anemia (pale skin, fatigue), constipation, breathing difficulties. Many suffer from iron deficiency. |
| Potassium | Vegetables, fruits, whole grains, legumes. | Fluid balance, nervous system, controls activities of heart, muscle, and kidneys. | Poor reflexes, irregular heartbeat, dry skin, general weakness. |
| Magnesium | Nuts, green vegetables, whole grains, seafood. | Acid/alkaline balance, important in metabolism of carbohydrates, minerals, and sugar. | Nervousness, tremors, easily aroused anger, disorientation, blood clots. |
| Copper | Oysters, nuts, legumes. | Formation of red blood cells, bone growth and health. Works with vitamin C to form elastin. | General weakness, impaired respiration, skin sores. |

| | BEST SOURCE | FUNCTION | DEFICIENCY SYMPTOMS |
|---|---|---|---|
| Iodine | Seafood, seaweed, salt. | Component of hormone thyroxine which controls metabolism. | Goiter, dry skin and hair, nervousness, obesity. |
| Phosphorus | Fish, meat, poultry, eggs, grains. | Bone development, important protein, fat, carbohydrate utilization. | Poor bones and teeth. Arthritis, appetite loss, irregular breathing, rickets. |
| Zinc | Eggs, lean meats, seafood, whole grains. | Aid in hearing, involved in digestion and metabolism. Important in development of reproductive system. | Retarded growth, prolonged wound healing, loss of appetite. |
| Selenium | Seafood, lean meats, grains. | Protects body tissue against oxidative damage from radiation, pollution and normal metabolic processing. | Heart muscle abnormalities. |

Source: AICR, Complete Eater's Digest and Nutrition Scoreboard by Michael F. Jacobson, Ph.D. Nutrition Almanac; John Kirschman, director

# FOOD SAFETY

Food poisoning is the top item on the list of food hazards. Health officials agree that the processing, preparation, and distribution of food are monitored very effectively, but that consumers and cooks must be knowledgeable about and obey the rules of proper preparation and proper storage to protect themselves and their families against the danger of food poisoning.

Each year, some two million Americans suffer food poisoning, according to the U.S. Department of Agriculture (USDA). In most cases, poisoning could have been prevented by the proper handling of food in the home or food-service establishments. Salmonella infection alone is estimated to affect more than a million people each year in the United States. Salmonella is hardest on the very young and the very old, and can kill, cripple, or leave its victim with a serious health problem. Salmonella is also resistant to antibiotics. Anyone who is involved in food preparation and handling needs to know as much as possible about the prevention of food-borne illnesses.

A USDA seal on raw meat or poultry does not guarantee that it is free of potentially harmful bacteria. The seal only shows that the meat has been inspected for quality. Chicken and holiday turkeys are the most frequently named carriers of salmonella bacteria, but salmonella can be passed on by virtually any uncooked meat, eggs, raw milk, even feces of dogs, cats, turtles, and humans.

After purchasing the product, it is vitally important to handle it in such a way that the bacteria present will not cause food poisoning. Not only can the food be contaminated when we purchase it, but we can transmit bacteria to the food. Unwashed hands can carry fecal bacteria to foods. Bacteria of the skin, hair, nose, and throat can cause food poisoning as the result of coughing, sneezing, or just touching foods. If we take a contaminated food home, cut it up on the cutting board, and cook it, we will kill the bacteria in that food. BUT some cooks might continue preparing a salad, for example, without washing hands, cutting board, or knife, and thus introduce salmonella into the salad. The salad eaters then may or may not develop salmonellosis. This is called cross-contamination, and can also occur when, for example, you barbecue a steak and return it to the same unwashed platter or cutting board that held it when it was raw.

*Salmonella* — Named for Daniel Salmon, a microbiologist who isolated it 100 years ago. Salmonella COMMONLY does not infect fruits, vegetables, or salmon.

*Staphylococcus Aureus* — Microbes that are found on human skin, and are the most common cause of food-borne illness in the United States. The toxin produced by staphylococcus aureus is resistant to heat and retains the ability to cause illness even though the germ is dead.

*Clostridium Botulism* — Produces a toxin so deadly that one teaspoon could kill five million people. Botulism is rare, but when it strikes, it is deadly. Botulism toxin is destroyed by high heat.

## FOOD SAFETY RULES

*To prevent illness from SALMONELLA:*
- Do not thaw meats or poultry at room temperature. Instead, thaw overnight in the refrigerator or use cold running water, changing the water often, or thaw in a microwave oven.
- Do not leave hot foods at room temperature or at a warm holding temperature for more than two hours.
- Refrigerate leftovers promptly. Do not cool on kitchen counter, and reheat thoroughly before serving again. If storing large amounts, divide into smaller portions that can cool more rapidly to a safe temperature.

*AVOID CROSS-CONTAMINATION* by using hot, soapy water to clean hands, utensils, cutting boards, or counter tops that have been in contact with raw meat, poultry, fish, eggs, and raw milk.
- When stuffing a turkey, do so just before cooking. (It is best to cook stuffing separately.) Use a meat thermometer to avoid undercooking. Cook to an internal temperature of 190°. Insert thermometer between the thigh and the body of the bird, making sure

the thermometer tip is not touching the bone. (If not using a thermometer, allow 20 minutes per pound up to six pounds and 15 minutes per pound for larger birds. In both cases add 5 minutes per pound if stuffed.)
- Do not use hands to mix foods. Keep hands away from hair, nose, and mouth when handling foods. A person with a skin infection or infectious disease should not be handling food.

*To prevent illness from CLOSTRIDIUM BOTULISM:*
- Obtain reliable canning instructions, available from the USDA.
- Use only the pressure canner method of canning vegetables, meats, and poultry. The high temperatures needed to kill botulism bacteria cannot be reached by other home canning methods, except in the case of a few fruits and pickled vegetables that are sufficiently acidic to prevent bacterial growth and toxin formation. These may be canned in a hot water bath. If in doubt about the home canning procedure used, boil meat, poultry, corn, or spinach for 20 minutes, and at least 10 minutes for other vegetables. Do not taste food you suspect.

*TIPS:*
- Pick up perishable foods last at the market and get them home and refrigerated quickly. Do not leave your groceries in the car while running errands.
- Do not buy products stored above the frost line in the store freezers.
- Do not buy products that appear to be tampered with or opened.
- Most food poisoning bacteria are killed at cooking temperatures between 165° and 212°. For red meat 140° is recommended, and for pork, between 165-170°. These temperatures are internal temperatures recorded on a meat thermometer.
- Keep your refrigerator set at 40° or lower.
- Leave store wrapping on food when refrigerating, if not torn. Repeated handling can introduce bacteria. However, when freezing chicken it is advisable to remove it from the store tray, wash, pat dry, and re-wrap it.

- Do not interrupt cooking since this may encourage bacteria growth before cooking is completed.
- Allow one and one-half times more cooking time for frozen foods than you use for cooking similar thawed foods. (Does not apply to microwave cooking.)
- Maintain a CLEAN kitchen that is free of flies and insects. Wash or replace those dirty, crumbling sponges and grimy towels. Clean up food spills and crumb-filled crevices. Hot, soapy water will immobilize bacteria and wash them away. Cold water will not!
- Wood cutting boards are not recommended for cutting meats and poultry because bacteria can enter cracks in the wood, and careful washing may not remove them.

*Sources:*
1. *AICR Newsletter, spring 1986, issue II.*
2. *Nutrition Action Health Letter, volume 13, number 6, June 1986.*
3. *Understanding Nutrition 4E, Whitney & Hamilton, Food Poisoning.*

## IS IT REALLY CHEESE?

High-fat natural cheeses are among the pitfalls in a diet to lower cancer risk. However, with a little extra knowledge about cheese and some of its imitators, you can still indulge.

The natural or aged cheeses — including cheddar, gouda, havarti, roquefort, and swiss — are made from whole milk and may be enriched with cream. They may naturally contain 8-10 grams of fat per ounce of cheese — about the same as well marbled red meat — and at least 75 percent of the calories in these cheeses is contributed by fat.

The milkfat provides flavor, texture and overall appeal to the hard cheeses and, until recently, lower fat versions were disliked for being rubbery, dry, and tasteless. With advances in food technology, today's varieties of imitation cheeses are much more appealing.

By definition, imitation cheese contains less butterfat than required by the Standards of Identity for natural cheese; they may contain ingredients not specified in the Standards. For instance, some of the low-cholesterol products replace butterfat with vegetable oil. There is less cholesterol and saturated fat, but the TOTAL fat content is unchanged — you must look closely at the ingredients on the label. Watch out for "low-sodium" and "lite" versions; many times the only difference is the reduction of salt, not fat. Also check the nutrient content. Some imitation cheeses are significantly lower in certain dairy food nutrients than the original natural cheese. (Beware, nutritional information does not always appear on the cheese wrappers because the Food and Drug Administration sets standards which a product must meet to be called a "cheese." The FDA specifies types and amounts of ingredients, minimum percentages of fat, maximum moisture content, pasteurization or ripening requirements, and product procedures. Since the standards are published in the Code of Federal Regulations, they need not appear on the label. Manufacturers frequently DO include ingredient information for health-conscious consumers, but the labeling is not mandatory.)

When surveying the dairy case, note that cheese products labeled as "lowfat" are generally lowest in fat. But those labeled "reduced fat" or "part-skim" can also be good choices. Check the label. Choose those that contain no more than 4 grams of fat per ounce of cheese (or per $1/2$ cup of cottage or ricotta cheese). The lowest fat cheeses have at least three times as many grams of protein as grams of fat. (There is very little carbohydrate in cheese.) If you cannot find lowfat cheeses in your favorite supermarket, suggest to the store manager that the store carry them. If there is enough demand, the store will do so. Lowfat cheeses can be substituted for their high-fat counterparts in recipes without much difficulty. You will find some differences in texture and melting qualities but continue cooking with these cheeses and you will benefit in the long run. Use the following list as a guide when shopping for lowfat cheeses.

| Lowfat Cheeses | Medium-Fat Cheeses | High-Fat Cheeses |
|---|---|---|
| (1 gram fat/oz. [weight] or ¼ cup [volume]) | (6 gram fat/oz.) | (8 gram fat/oz. or ¼ cup) |
| Cottage-dry curd<br>Cottage 1%<br>   2% milkfat<br>Gammelmost<br>Mysost<br>Primost<br>Ricotta | Cheezola<br>Feta<br>Pasteurized processed<br>   cheese spread | Blue          Limberger<br>Brie          Longhorn<br>Brick          Parmesan<br>Edam          Port du Salut<br>Gjetost          Swiss<br>Provolone          Whole-milk<br>Romano          ricotta<br>Gouda |
| (2-4 grams fat/oz. or ¼ cup) | (7 grams fat/oz.) | (9 grams fat/oz.) |
| Baker's<br>Cottage-4% milkfat<br>Dorman's Low-Chol™<br>Farmer<br>Hoop<br>Schreiber Cheese Food<br>Laughing Cow™<br>Light & Lively™<br>Lite Line™<br>Weight Watchers™<br>St. Otho Swiss<br>Whole milk mozzarella | Camembert<br>Dorman-Slim Jack™<br>Liederkranz<br>Neufchatel<br>Tilsit | American<br>Cheddar<br>Colby<br>Gorgonzola<br>Gruyere<br>Monterey Jack<br>Muenster |
| (5 grams fat/oz. or ¼ cup) | | (10 grams fat/oz.) |
| Part-skim mozzarella<br>Part-skim ricotta<br>Pot cheese<br>Sapsago | | Cream cheese |

*Source: American Institute for Cancer Research, Winter 1988 Newsletter, Issue 18.*

# WHAT IS OSTEOPOROSIS?

Osteoporosis is a condition in which bone tissue decreases. As bones become thinner, they become more fragile and porous and are therefore more susceptible to fracture. A fall, blow, or lifting action, which would not bruise or strain the average person, can easily break a bone in someone with severe osteoporosis. Disabilities from such fractures are often the beginning of serious physical decline for elderly people.

**WHO IS AT RISK?** — The disorder of osteoporosis is eight times greater in women than in men, partly because women have less bone mass to start with. Rarely, osteoporosis may strike a person who is only in her mid-thirties, but in most cases the patient is in her fifties or sixties when the disorder is diagnosed. Women who have passed menopause are especially vulnerable, apparently because changes in the body's hormone levels accelerate loss of bone tissue. At greatest risk of osteoporosis are women who 1) are approaching menopause or passing through it or who are past menopause; 2) have recently had surgical removal of the ovaries; 3) have a family history of osteoporosis in their mothers, aunts, or sisters. Black women are at much lower risk of suffering from this disorder because they tend to have greater bone mass. Hip fractures, for example, are three times more common among white women than among black women. In general, small-boned Caucasian and Oriental women are most susceptible to osteoporosis.

**WHAT CAUSES OSTEOPOROSIS?** — Living bone contains a soft protein framework in which calcium salts are deposited. Calcium gives bone its familiar hardness. Bone, like other body tissues, is constantly being rebuilt or remodeled. Old bone is torn down, reabsorbed by the body, and replaced with new bone in much the same way that people remodel buildings by tearing out new walls and replacing them with new structures. As a person gets older, the amount of the bone replaced during normal remodeling falls increasingly short of the amount reabsorbed. By age 35 or 40, both men and women have begun to lose some bone material. By the time a person reaches her mid-sixties, the body's ability to absorb calcium from

**50**

food begins to deteriorate, further aggravating net bone loss. Several other factors also contribute to bone breakdown: Menopause, a family history of osteoporosis, a sedentary lifestyle, immoderate alcohol consumption, cigarette smoking, and too little calcium in the diet. Additional factors that can contribute to bone loss include: Certain drugs, such as cortisone, and heparin; disorders such as hyperthyroidism and kidney disease; impaired ability to absorb calcium from the intestines; excessive excreation of calcium in the urine; increased demand for calcium during pregnancy and lactation; and certain foods taken in excess, such as protein.

**WHAT ARE THE SYMPTOMS?** — Generally people with osteoporosis have no pain or other symptoms until their bones become so weak that a sudden strain, bump, or fall causes a fracture. Often the condition is discovered on an X-ray taken for some other purpose. Another clue to the presence of osteoporosis, even if there is no pain, is loss of height. Some people do have pain, however, either a chronic aching along the spine or pain from spasm in the muscles of the back.

**HOW CAN OSTEOPOROSIS BE PREVENTED?** — Osteoporosis is so common that all women should consider adopting lifestyle habits that will protect their bones, particularly adequate dietary intake of calcium and regular weight-bearing exercise, such as walking or running. A woman should get plenty of calcium in her diet throughout life — but particularly after age 40. In childhood and adolescence and before menopause, 800 milligrams of calcium is probably sufficient. (This is also recommended daily amount for men.) Pregnancy and lactating women require an additional 500 milligrams. After menopause, the requirement for women increases to more than 1,000 milligrams (1 gram) per day. So doctors recommend between 1,000 and 3,000 milligrams per day, especially for women who are not taking estrogen.

*Sources:*

*1. OSTEOPOROSIS, cause, treatment, prevention. Prepared by: National Institute of Arthritis, Diabetes, and Digestive and Kidney Diseases. Published by U.S. Department of Health and Human Services, Public Health Services, National Institutes of Health.*

*2. American Institute for Cancer Research, 1987 Newsletter, Osteoporosis/Calcium Update.*

# PLEASE PASS THE CALCIUM

Calcium is the mineral that gives bones their strength and hardness. Without calcium, our bones would be so soft that they could be bent and tied into knots. But merely getting enough calcium is not sufficient to keep bones strong. Although calcium is important, a nutritional balancing act is required for maintaining strong bones.

The current Recommended Dietary Allowance (RDA) of calcium

## CALCIUM AND FAT CONTENT

| Food | Amount | Calcium (milligrams) | Fat (grams) |
|---|---|---|---|
| **Milk and Dairy Products** | | | |
| American cheese | 1 oz. | 174 mg. | 8.9 g. |
| Cheddar cheese | 1 oz. | 204 mg. | 9.4 g. |
| Cottage cheese, creamed | 1 cup | 126 mg. | 9.5 g. |
| Mozzarella cheese, part-skim | 1 oz. | 195 mg. | 4.7 g. |
| Swiss cheese | 1 oz. | 272 mg. | 7.8 g. |
| Ice cream, hard | 1 cup | 176 mg. | 14.3 g. |
| Whole milk | 1 cup | 291 mg. | 8.2 g. |
| Lowfat milk (2%) | 1 cup | 297 mg. | 4.7 g. |
| Skim milk | 1 cup | 302 mg. | 0.4 g. |
| Lowfat plain yogurt | 1 cup | 415 mg. | 3.5 g. |
| Lowfat plain yogurt with fruit | 1 cup | 345 mg. | 2.4 g. |
| Ricotta cheese, part-skim | ½ cup | 337 mg. | 9.8 g. |
| **Green Leafy Vegetables** | | | |
| Broccoli, cooked | 1 cup | 178 mg. | 0.4 g. |
| Kale, cooked without stem | 1 cup | 178 mg. | 0.6 g. |
| Spinach, cooked | 1 cup | 244 mg. | 0.5 g. |
| Turnip greens, cooked | 1 cup | 198 mg. | 0.3 g. |
| **Other Vegetables** | | | |
| Beans, canned with pork and tomato | ½ cup | 68 mg. | 3.2 g. |
| Beans, green snap, cooked | 1 cup | 58 mg. | 0.4 g. |
| Chickpeas, garbanzos, canned | 3½ oz. | 75 mg. | 2.4 g. |
| Soybeans, cooked | ½ cup | 131 mg. | 5.8 g. |
| Sweet potato, baked in skin | 1 small | 40 mg. | 0.5 g. |

for adults is 800 milligrams, but there is disagreement about how much calcium the body really needs. All agree, however, that the body does need calcium.

Dairy products are good sources of calcium, and lowfat dairy products make it possible to get enough calcium without gaining weight. Other sources of the mineral are dark green and leafy vegetables like collards, turnip greens, spinach, and broccoli. While some

## OF COMMON FOODS

| Food | Amount | Calcium (milligrams) | Fat (grams) |
|---|---|---|---|
| **Nuts** | | | |
| Almonds, roasted and salted | ¼ cup | 91.8 mg. | 22.6 g. |
| Sesame seeds, dried, hulled | ¼ cup | 40 mg. | 17.6 g. |
| Sunflower seeds, dry roasted | ¼ cup | 22 mg. | 15.9 g. |
| **Seafood** | | | |
| Sardines, in oil, drained* | 3 oz. | 372 mg. | 9.0 g. |
| Scallops, steamed | 3½ oz. | 115 mg. | 1.4 g. |
| Shrimp, raw | 3½ oz. | 63 mg. | 0.8 g. |
| Salmon, canned* | 3½ oz. | 249 mg. | 5.2 g. |
| **Other Foods** | | | |
| Bread, white or whole wheat | 2 slices | 46 mg. | 2.0 g. |
| Candy, milk chocolate bar | 1 oz. | 64 mg. | 9.0 g. |
| Chili con carne with beans | 5 oz. | 61 mg. | 9.9 g. |
| Cream of celery soup, made with milk | 1 serving | 135 mg. | 33.0 g. |
| Figs, dried | 5 med. | 126 mg. | 1.3 g. |
| Orange, raw | 1 med. | 56 mg. | 0.1 g. |
| Pizza, cheese, 12-inch slice | 1 piece | 144 mg. | 4.4 g. |
| Pudding, chocolate, cornstarch | ½ cup | 147 mg. | 6.6 g. |
| Raisins, dried, seedless | ⅝ cup | 62 mg. | 0.2 g. |
| Tofu | 4 oz. | 154 mg. | 5.0 g. |
| Waffles, plain, enriched | 1 med. | 85 mg. | 7.4 g. |

*The bones of sardines and salmon must be eaten to get the full calcium value.

*Source: American Institute for Cancer Research*

leafy greens contain oxalic acid, which can theoretically interfere with the body's use of calcium, its effect is not important in the portions usually eaten. Salmon, sardines, oysters, nuts, and tofu (soybean curd) also contain calcium. The chart on pages 52 and 53 should help in the choice of calcium-rich foods that are not high in fat.

Certain lifestyle habits may increase the requirement for calcium. Cigarette smoking, alcohol, and foods and drinks containing caffeine, such as coffee and chocolate, increase calcium requirement, and should be avoided by those concerned with calcium deficiency.

Eating large amounts of protein may also cause calcium loss through the urine. The Recommended Dietary Allowance for protein is 48 grams per day for adult women and 56 grams per day for adult men. There is no scientific basis for suggesting that much more than this is necessary, although to be assured of this amount, regularly consuming 60-70 grams per day is probably harmless. One serving of cottage cheese (4 ounces) contains 14 grams of protein. Three slices of turkey contain about 31 grams of protein.

Another part of the balancing act is vitamin D. The body must have this vitamin in order to absorb calcium (the RDA for vitamin D is 400 IU). One cup of fortified milk has 100 IU of vitamin D; egg yolk, saltwater fish, and liver are other good sources. The best way to get vitamin D, however, is fifteen minutes to an hour of midday sunshine, since adequate amounts of the vitamin are produced in the exposed skin. Because vitamin D is produced in this way, it is now considered to be a hormone, not a vitamin. None needs to be consumed if one has adequate sunshine.

Finally, a brief word about fiber. Too much of anything is not advisable, and too much fiber can prevent the body from absorbing calcium. See pages 33 through 36, Fiber's Role in Good Health.

## STIR-FRY

Stir-frying is easy and fast, and the results are extremely delicious. As an added bonus, it is also healthy and recommended eating by the American Institute of Cancer Research. Wok cooking is gaining in popularity for many reasons, foremost among them being rapid preparation, using very little cooking oil. As little as one Tablespoon of oil is needed to create a deliciously healthy meal for several people. The variety of foods you can use is endless. Leftovers are transformed when "wokked." The trick to stir-frying is organization.

**GETTING READY:**
- Read the recipe well.
- If using dried foods (seaweed, mushrooms, etc.), allow for soaking time, usually 20-30 minutes.
- Prepare seafood or poultry according to recipe (removing skin or shells, slicing, chopping, etc.). This may be done ahead of time, then covered and refrigerated for later use. Marinate if called for.
- Prepare vegetables for cooking. Remember to keep vegetables as dry as possible to prevent splattering in hot oil. Keep in mind the cooking times for various vegetables. Separate the slow-cooking from the quick-cooking vegetables.
- Mix liquid seasonings unless recipe specifies otherwise, and organize remaining ingredients such as ginger, onions, garlic, garnish, etc. Having everything cut up and ready is the key.

Set up wok, set stabilizing ring over burner and place wok on top of it — GET SET, GO!

1. Heat wok and oil.
2. Add seasonings — garlic, onions, ginger, etc.
3. Add meats, poultry, or seafood, and the slow-cooking vegetables.
4. Add liquid seasonings.
5. Add quick-cooking vegetables.
6. Add paste (if called for) or liquid seasonings.

Stir constantly over medium or medium-high heat until meats and vegetables are done.

55

## SNACKING

If you are a closet eater, between-meal snacker, or midnight muncher, you can rid yourself of your guilty feelings by learning how to snack. Snacking can be good for you and still be satisfying. It depends WHAT you choose to snack on, and what you make available for your family to snack on.

Get rid of the soda pop, the salted nuts, the Twinkies. Forget the greasy potato chips and the double-fudge brownies! Avoid the supermarket aisles where these temptations lurk if you cannot resist buying them.

Instead, choose high-fiber, lowfat, low-calorie foods and LEARN to think of them as goodies.

Fruit is an excellent snack food — high in fiber and vitamins, and low in cholesterol, it will help eliminate the sweetness craving and will give you the added "pick up" you need. If you are in the apple, orange, banana rut, check over the fruit section, starting on page 301 for some new ideas. Make small fruit salads with seasonal fruits and keep them handy. There will be little waste, little preparation time, and you can offer a variety every few days. Another way I promote fruit is by keeping a bowl of a variety of fresh fruits out on the kitchen counter, where it catches the eye, instead of in the crisper (out of sight, out of mind).

Vegetables are a valuable snack. They provide vitamins, fiber, and no cholesterol. Try keeping a container of carrot and celery sticks, bell pepper strips, mushrooms, and other colorful veggies in the refrigerator, readily available to the snacker. For some ideas, look over the vegetable section starting on page 73.

Popcorn (without the extras) is a perfect low-calorie, high-fiber food, and it is fun to eat. Crackers and lowfat cheese are another good combo.

According to the American Institute for Cancer Research, judicious snacking keeps your blood sugar level and your "pep quotient" balanced throughout the day, and provides you with a better variety of healthy foods.

56

## WATER: THE NECESSARY NUTRIENT

Getting enough water is as important to our bodies as getting enough food. Our cells, which are composed mainly of water, couldn't even function without enough water in them. Did you know that our bodies are about two-thirds water? The water does a lot of "work" each day. The water in our mouths softens food when we eat and makes it easier to swallow. The water in the stomach mixes with food and helps the digestive process. And once the food is digested and absorbed, our blood (consisting mostly of water) carries the nutrients to the cells and transports waste products away. Water is also the body's thermostat. Each day our bodies lose about two quarts of water. In hot weather, we can lose three quarts. When exercising vigorously, or just walking on a very warm day, our bodies will cool off through perspiration. If you are thirsty, it probably means your body needs more water. Since water plays such an important role, make sure you are getting the equivalent of six to eight glasses of water each day. Remember that fresh fruits and vegetables contain a high percentage of water.

## BARBECUING TIPS

There is little evidence that Americans are at risk from excessive charcoal broiled foods, according to the American Institute of Cancer Research (AICR). Much remains to be learned about how this popular cooking method produces cancer-causing agents in our foods.

While researchers search for answers, MODERATION in consumption is highly recommended by AICR. The following are barbecuing guidelines to healthy eating:

- Reduce the amount of meat you consume. Since high levels of fat and protein found in meat may be associated with increased risk of cancer, the amount of meat you eat can be as important as how you cook it.

- Select meats that are low in fat. Research shows that the higher the level of fat in charcoal-broiled meats, the greater the production of carcinogens.
- Try covering the grill with aluminum foil before you cook out. Holes can be punched between the grids to let fat drip out. The foil will protect food from smoke and the fire.
- Trim excess fat before cooking.
- Substitute fish or poultry (with skin and fat removed) for more fatty meats.
- When grilling fish, select one of the leaner fish. Besides having less fat, it will hold its shape better during cooking.
- Cook meat until it is done WITHOUT charring it.
- Remove any charred material that does form on the food's surface.
- Avoid tendency to overcook.
- Discourage flare ups. Burning juice or fat adds nothing to the charcoal flavor of foods, but can produce harmful smoke.
- Keep a squirt bottle of water handy for dampening coals that become too hot or flare up.
- If smoke from dripping fat is too heavy, move the food to another section of the grill, rotate grill, or reduce the heat.
- Some foods, especially fish and vegetables, can be cooked on a grill in foil to protect them.
- When fat from meat drips onto the hot coals or stones, it forms a substance (benzopyrene) that is identified as a carcinogen. The smoke that then rises from the fire carries this substance back up to the meat and deposits it on the surface of the food.

## BARBECUING

Ignite the coals and allow the fire to burn down completely before cooking — about 20 minutes. Do not squirt starting fluid over burning coals.

Levels of heat needed will be dictated by the type of food. There are three levels:

*Hot Coals* — Coals barely covered with gray ash and may have a low flame.

58

*Medium Coals* — Coals well covered with ash and may have a glow.

*Low Coals* — Coals completely covered with a thick layer of ash.

## Turkey

Never stuff a turkey when barbecuing it; cooking is slow and keeps the stuffing at an unsafe temperature for too long, creating a danger of salmonella contamination.

Whole turkey can be barbecued in a covered pan 15-20 minutes per pound over hot coals.

If using a rotisserie, cook for 30 minutes per pound. The meat thermometer should register 180°.

## Pork

*Chops* — One inch thickness cook 35-40 minutes, turning twice.

*Roasts* — Use rotisserie and a meat thermometer to 170°. A 4-5 pound roast will require 1 hour to reach well done.

*Leg* — Takes longer than a roast because of its larger diameter. Cook 35-40 minutes per pound.

## Seafood

Fish with firm textures such as salmon, red snapper, halibut, cod, or swordfish do best on the barbecue in steaks or fillets. Allow 10 minutes per inch of thickness.

*Whole Trout* — Grill 4-6 inches from coals, allowing 12 minutes per inch of thickness.

*Prawns* — Place on a skewer and grill 4-6 inches from hot coals, turning often and basting with a favorite sauce or garlic butter until prawns are pink, about 3 minutes.

## Lamb

*Butterflied Leg of Lamb* — 30-45 minutes over medium coals, turn frequently.

*Chops, Ribs, Shoulders* — 10-12 minutes over medium coals, turn once during cooking.

*Roasts* — Use meat thermometer, cook to internal temperature of 145-150° for rare, and 170° for well.

## Chicken

Barbecued chicken is my daughter's absolute favorite. Whole birds, halves, breasts, legs or thighs all taste great and are excellent in take-along lunches.

Remove the skin and extra fat, cover with favorite sauce, and marinate until ready to cook. Turn chicken often for even browning (every 10 minutes), brushing with marinade. Chicken will cook in 45 minutes to 1 hour depending on size, while a 4-pound chicken on a rotisserie will require 2-2½ hours over medium coals. Insert meat thermometer into the thickest part of the thigh — temperature should reach 180°.

*Chicken Breasts* — Cook 10-12 minutes per pound over medium coals.

*Thighs and Drumsticks* — Wrap in foil for first part of cooking to keep tender and moist. Brush with marinade.

Turn chicken with tongs rather than a fork so as not to lose juices.

For more information contact the American Institute of Cancer Research, Washington, D.C. 20069-2012.

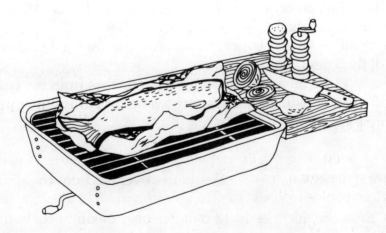

# SPICES AND HERBS

**Allspice** — This spice is delicious in cakes, cookies, breads, fruit salads, and even pickles. Allspice is an individual spice, not a combination of spices as its name suggests. It is the dried, pea-sized fruit of a pimiento tree that grows in Mexico, Jamaica, and Central and South America. The flavor is comparable to a mixture of cinnamon, nutmeg, and cloves. Allspice can be bought whole or ground.

**Anise** — Has a licorice flavor that tastes great in cookies, breads, candies, and tea. It can be purchased ground or whole (anise stars). The anise plant needs full sun.

**Basil** — "The tomato herb," basil has a robust, marvelous flavor and smell. Noted for its affinity for tomatoes, used in stews, soups, spaghetti, seafood, pasta, pesto, vegetables, eggs, and excellent in salads. ½ teaspoon dried = 1 Tablespoon fresh. The basil plant will tolerate light shade.

**Bay Leaf** — Bay leaves (the dried leaves of a laurel tree) have a pungent flavor that keeps very well. Bay leaf is essential in bouquet garni, pot roasts, beans, paté, soups, corned beef, also used with chicken, lamb, and bland vegetables.

**Bouquet Garni** — Usually composed of parsley, bay leaf and thyme tied together with a string or enclosed in cheesecloth. It is used to flavor soups, stew, and braised meats. If you desire you can also add celery leaves, peppercorns, lemon or orange rinds, basil, chervil, rosemary, or tarragon. The reason for tying the herbs together is to make it easy to remove the bouquet garni before serving.

**Caraway Seed** — A flavor that combines anise and dill. A spiky seed, caraway has many uses — tossed in a salad or noodles, added to breads and cookies, cooked with sauerkraut, or added to cheese.

**Cardamom** — Whole or ground, used in baking. Strongly spicy, resembling cloves and lemon peel — use sparingly!

**61**

**Chervil** — Chervil resembles parsley, but the flavor is more subtle. Add fresh leaves to salads or use as a garnish. Chervil is especially good with chicken, fish, and egg dishes.

**Chili Powder** — Made from dried chilies, commercial chili powder is mildly hot, self ground chili is hotter, so use with caution.

**Chives** — Chives belong to the onion family. Use fresh whenever possible for a mild onion flavor and crunchiness. When fresh chives are not available, try freeze-dried. Use with almost any food — soups, fish, seafood, vegetables, dips, sour cream. Chives are great for kitchen gardens. Plant is less than one foot tall and prefers full sun.

**Cinnamon** — Ground cinnamon is used in many desserts, main dishes, stews, French toast or waffles, bread, rolls, rice, apple dishes, and jams. The list is endless. Hot chocolate. . . .

**Cloves** — Nail-shaped flower bud of an evergreen tree, belonging to the myrtle family. Ground cloves are used in baking cakes, breads, and cookies. Whole cloves can be used in a variety of ways: studded on baked ham, in pickling spices, stuck into an onion or wrapped in cheesecloth for stews and soups. Cloves have a sweet, pungent flavor. Try making a pomander ball for your closet (or as a traditional Christmas gift) by sticking cloves all over an orange.

**Coriander or Cilantro** — The fresh leaves of the coriander plant are known as cilantro, or Mexican or Chinese parsley. The leaves have a surprisingly unfamiliar taste, and are used frequently in Mexican, Indian, and Chinese cooking. Cilantro is delicious in salsa, salads, and lasagne; try using it in pesto instead of basil for a tasty surprise. Coriander seeds are essential in pickling, and ground coriander seeds are used as a spice in baking. The coriander plant will survive in a shady area.

**Curry** — Curry is not a single spice, but a blend of spices including turmeric, cumin, coriander, fenugreek, red pepper, and others. It can actually contain as many as 16-20 spices. Curry is an essential ingredient in Indian cooking. It is used in stews, salad dressings, sauces, eggs, vegetables, fish, lamb, and rice. Use cautiously because blends vary in strength.

**Dill** — A member of the parsley family. Fresh dill is more flavorful than dried, and is available in most markets when in season. Use in salads, soups, vegetables, and pickling. Salmon and dill are a delicious combination. Also use in cottage cheese, sour cream, and potatoes. Even though dill has a mild flavor, it can be overwhelming when used with a heavy hand. Dill is a tall growing plant, preferring full sun. 1 teaspoon dried = 1 Tablespoon fresh. Dill is too delicate to freeze.

**Dry Mustard** — Dry ground mustard is made from mustard seeds. It is strong, so use very little as directed.

**Fennel** — Fennel seed has a licorice flavor. If you use too much it can be bitter. It is an essential ingredient in many Italian dishes. Try in breads, fish, chicken, even tofu dishes. The fennel bulb is a delicious vegetable, unfamiliar to many. Check vegetable section on page 84.

**Fenugreek** — Smells like celery but has a bitter flavor. Used in many African dishes, and delicious in curries.

**Filé** — Powdered sassafras leaf, used in stews, soups, and with seafood. Filé is a necessary ingredient of creole gumbos. It should be added to an already hot dish and not allowed to boil.

**Garden Burnet** — A little known spring herb that has an aromatic smell, which makes a pleasant addition to salads.

**Ginger** — Ginger is now available in almost any market in many forms. You may find the gray-white bulb peeled, or the root, or powdered or candied ginger. The upper stems of the ginger plant grow 3-4 feet high. After they wither, the roots are dug up and dried. Ginger root is a natural ingredient that enhances the flavor of many foods, and can be used freshly grated, sliced, pickled, or candied. It is superb with chicken, fish, seafood, and vegetables, in marinades, and is an essential ingredient in Chinese cooking. Fresh ginger will keep about a week refrigerated, or grate it and freeze for use as needed. Ground ginger is used mainly in baking.

**Juniper Berries** — These berries have the aromatic flavor that gives gin its distinctive taste. Use in tea, meat marinades, and sauces.

**Mace** — Mace is the outer covering of nutmeg, with a milder flavor than nutmeg. Found dried or ground. Used most often in baking.

**Marjoram (sweet)** — This versatile herb is a member of the mint family, but is often confused with oregano. Marjoram has a sweeter, more delicate flavor. Because of its delicate flavor, it should be added to cooked dishes toward the end of the cooking time. Marjoram is great in almost any dish. Like basil, it has an affinity for tomatoes. Is also good with lamb, chicken, liver, soups, sauces, and pizza. When dried, it loses its flavor quickly, so purchase small amounts. $1/2$ teaspoon dried = 1 Tablespoon fresh. Marjoram grows to a height of 1-2 feet, and produces pink and purple blooms, preferring a sunny spot.

**Mint** — Use as a fresh, pretty garnish for summer drinks. Tossed with potatoes, baked with lamb roast, or steeped with tea, mint is very refreshing. The plant likes full sun, but will tolerate partial shade, and spreads like wildfire!

**Nutmeg** — Buy whole nutmeg and grate it fresh to give a wonderful, fragrant taste and aroma to certain vegetables (especially cauliflower), cakes, cookies, stews, and hot chocolate. When grating, use the smallest holes on your grater, or purchase a special grater for nutmeg. Of course, you can also buy ground nutmeg.

**Oregano** — This herb enhances most dishes, from stuffings and stews, to poultry, lamb, seafood, vegetables, dips, pizza, and pasta. Excellent in any tomato dish. The plant needs a sunny spot and makes an attractive houseplant.

**Paprika (sweet or hot)** — Many paprikas are very colorful but have no flavor. It pays to buy a quality paprika to enhance chicken and meat dishes, stews, and sauces.

**Parsley** — Parsley is considered an herb but its use as a vegetable is on the rise. It is an excellent source of vitamin A: 100 grams provide 5,200 IU of vitamin A. Parsley also provides some protein, calcium, potassium, folacin, with traces of vitamins and minerals. Available year round, with curly (the most popular) or flat (the more flavorful) leaves. There are at least 35 varieties of curly parsley. Parsley is a very flavorful addition to almost any recipe, and acts as a blending agent for other herbs. Parsley is also a useful breath freshener because of its power to destroy the scent of garlic and onions. Choose fresh green leaves, avoiding any that are yellow or wilted. Will keep about one week in refrigerator; wash when ready to use.

**Pickling Spice** — A combination of a variety of whole spices, such as mustard seed, cloves, ginger, coriander, cinnamon, bay leaf, dill, and peppers. Used in pickling, of course, but also in brine for fish. Try adding 2 Tablespoons to water when boiling prawns.

**Poppy Seed** — Poppy seeds have a crunchy, nut-like flavor. They are delicious in cakes, muffins, breads, cookies, salad dressings, and even tossed with pasta. I like to sprinkle poppy seeds on the tops of bread before baking. Poppy seeds are the seeds of a poppy plant.

**Rosemary** — For remembrance. Fresh rosemary is best, with a sweet, fresh taste. Use sparingly; it can easily overpower other herbs. Great with chicken, lamb, marinades, turkey, meatloaf, soups, and vegetable dishes. It is stiff-leaved, so chop, crumble or pulverize it thoroughly. 1/4 teaspoon dried = 1 teaspoon fresh. Plant prefers full sun. Plant in the garden in spring and bring indoors for winter use.

**Saffron** — Saffron is the stamen of the saffron crocus. Before using, saffron must be steeped in hot liquid to bring out its flavor. Buy it in its thread form rather than ground — the flavor will be fresher. Saffron gives a beautiful yellow color and very good flavor to chicken, lamb, rice, stews, and other dishes. Never use more than is called for.

**Sage** — Sage is very pungent, even when fresh. There are many kinds of sage: Aurea (variegated leaves), Purpurea (reddish purple leaves), and Albiflora (white flowers) are three of the many species. Also try "pineapple" sage for a fruity, aromatic flavor. Sage is primarily used in stuffings and sausage, but is also enjoyable with poultry, seafoods, biscuits, vegetables, and salads — and don't forget sage tea. Sage is a medium-size plant preferring full sun. Will tolerate partial sun, but flavor will be impaired.

**Sesame Seeds** — Have a sweet, nutty flavor. Sprinkle in or on anything. Toast seeds and toss over vegetables, soups, salads, breads. Give extra crunch to pan-fried fish or chicken, stir-fries, and cookies. Raw sesame seeds ground into a paste with nothing added is called Tahini or sesame seed butter, and can be found in most markets. Tahini can be used as a replacement for shortening in baking, or used in dressings. Experiment with it.

**Sorrel** (Sour Grass) — Has long stalks, and dark green leaves that resemble spinach. It has a sharp, sour lemon flavor and a high oxalic acid content. Can be cooked with spinach, but must be handled with care because sorrel will turn gray if cooked too hot or too long. If using in soups, add sorrel during the last 5 minutes of cooking so it will retain its color and flavor. Serve as a side dish or toss with greens in a salad. It also makes a refreshing iced tea.

**Tamarind** — Tamarind is a legume with large pods. When fully mature the pods are brown, a few inches long and about an inch wide. The brittle pod breaks away to reveal the brown pliable flesh that resembles fruit leather. This flesh covers a number of large shiny seeds. The fruit-leather flesh is the part used. Tamarind is high in carbohydrate, protein, minerals, and vitamin B-complex, with traces of vitamins A and C. Tamarind has a fruity, sour taste because of the tartaric acid it contains. Used in many Indian recipes. Great with chicken, curries, and preserves, and sometimes made into a candy

**66**

similar to fruit leather. To use break away outer skin and remove seeds. Now, either chop the leathery pulp and use it immediately, or pour boiling water over it, wait till it cools, then rub and squash the leathery pulp until it forms a paste. Use the paste as is or add pressed garlic to it for a very tasty mixture.

**Tarragon** — Tarragon is a beautiful herb with a delicate lemon licorice flavor. Especially good in fish, chicken, and vegetable dishes. Also try it in sauces, eggs, or mixed with vinegar. If not familiar with this herb, use sparingly at first. Tarragon is a medium-sized plant, preferring full sun.

**Thyme** — Thyme is a great herb for fish, seafood, lamb, beef, vegetables, poultry, pork, soups, stuffings, sauces, even tea. Remember to use small amounts as fresh thyme is a strong herb. Lemon enhances the flavor of thyme. Thyme is a low spreading plant and prefers full sun. $1/4$ teaspoon dried = 1 teaspoon fresh.

**Lemon Thyme** — Great in salads and fish and chicken recipes.

**White Pepper** — Black pepper and white pepper both come from the same plant, Piper Nigrum. To produce white pepper, the ripe berries have the skin and pulp removed. The inner white seeds are dried and ground.

**Capers** — Are small buds of a shrub grown in the Mediterranean. Can be purchased pickled, dried, or salted. The salted capers should be rinsed before using. Capers are superb with fish, sauces, salads, appetizers, and antipasto.

**Lemon Juice** — Fresh lemon juice enhances the flavor of most dishes and helps replace the need for salt. Use whenever possible in place of salt.

**Pimientos** — Are sweet red peppers preserved in oil. Use whole or chopped in salads, vegetable dishes, paté, or in meatloaf or rice dishes for added color.

**Pickapeppa** — Jamaican in origin. It is a very flavorful sauce. Ingredients are tomatoes, onions, raisins, mangos, tamarinds, and spices.

**Tabasco** — A hot liquid pepper flavoring. A few drops go a long way.

**Monosodium Glutamate** — Thought to be unhealthy. Many people have had physical reactions to it.

**Soy Sauce** — Is made from soybeans, wheat, salt, yeast, and sugar. Soy sauce is particularly good for marinating chicken and fish, or with rice, vegetables, and noodles. The low-sodium soy sauce is a healthy choice.

## *HELPFUL HINTS*

Stock — Ingredients should always be fresh and flavorful. Don't use the stock pot for foods that have been refrigerated too long and have lost their flavor. Season toward end of cooking. If you are going to store stock for later use, hold off salting until later.

Keep crackers crisp in the most humid weather by storing in the refrigerator. Be sure they are wrapped securely.

Honey — If it has crystallized, simply place the container of honey into a pot of boiling water.

Lemons — After squeezing the juice out of a lemon, wrap and freeze the rind. It's always on hand when you need fresh lemon rind.

If cream won't whip — Chill beaters and bowl or set bowl of cream in a bowl of ice while whipping. If you have no mixer, put cream into a tightly-lidded pint jar and shake. Check frequently so as not to overshake.

Cream whipped ahead of time will not separate if unflavored gelatin is added, $\frac{1}{4}$ teaspoon per cup of cream.

Avocados — Keep in brown paper bag or buried in a bowl of flour. Use a perforated plastic bag to promote ripening.

Brown sugar — Use a hand grater for sugar that is hard as a rock. If not needed right away, add a slice of soft bread to the package and close tightly. The sugar will soften within a few hours. You can also spread it out on a cookie tray and place in a 200° oven until the moisture dries out — keep checking.

Line refrigerator crisper (vegetable compartment) with paper towels. This will absorb excess moisture, helping fruits and vegetables keep longer (or you can use a small dry sponge to absorb excess moisture).

Try submerging a lemon in hot water for approximately 10 minutes. The lemon will yield almost twice the juice.

To keep fresh fruit from darkening after cutting, toss lightly with fresh lemon juice.

Freshen up cereal or crackers by putting them on a cookie sheet and heating in a moderate oven for about 10 minutes.

A leaf of lettuce dropped into a pot absorbs the grease from the top of soup. Remove the lettuce and throw away as soon as it has absorbed the grease.

Add a few teaspoons of cinnamon to an empty pie tin and slowly burn over the stove burner. Your kitchen will smell as though you have been baking all day.

Asparagus — Cut stalks diagonally and steam for 5-10 minutes, depending on size.

Pasta — Cook until almost done, then keep in a bowl of water. When needed, add to boiling water until done.

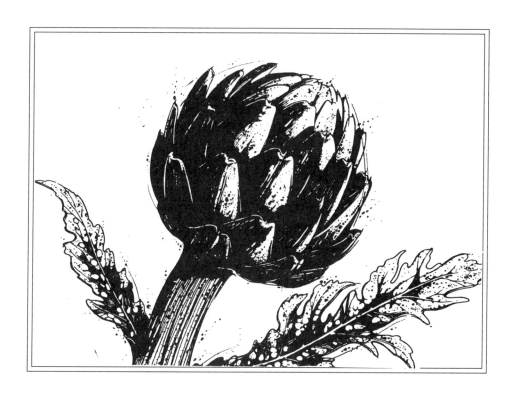

# VEGETABLES

## TAKE A WALK

According to most exercise physiologists, one of the best forms of exercise costs the least and is available to almost everyone — WALKING. A brisk walk after dinner helps stimulate circulation, aids digestion, and tones muscles. To increase aerobic benefits and upper body strength, carry light hand weights. Go alone, with a friend, or even the family dog. It is a great way to start or end the day!

Note: Use of excessive weights places added stress on bones and muscles and can result in a strain or sprain to knees, ankles, or back. If overweight, you already are stressing bones, muscles, tendons, as well as your back. If you are normal weight and are training for a specific goal such as a backpacking trip, practice hikes with added resistance can help.

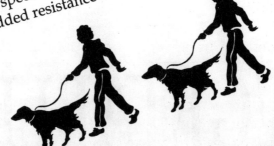

# VEGETABLES

When it comes to vegetables, Americans are deprived. Most of us stick to peas, carrots, cabbage, and corn. We ignore all the colorful and odd-shaped vegetables staring at us from the produce section. Fresh vegetables are remarkable: Virtually all are nutritious — some moderately, some extremely — and provide fiber, vitamins, minerals, and some protein. AICR* believes that fresh vegetables may help prevent cancer. Except for avocados and tomatoes, which are technically fruits, fresh vegetables contain virtually no fat and absolutely no cholesterol, are extremely low in sodium and calories, and have no sugar added, which all spells GOOD TO EAT.

We are fooled into believing that fast foods are nutritious, easy — and *fast*. The truth is that vegetables can be cooked in less than half the time needed for a T.V. dinner.

I have listed a wide variety of vegetables with a brief description of each, plus information on how to choose and store them. There are also some recipes to help you start adding more fresh vegetables to your diet. Good ways to experiment with new vegetables are in salads and stir-fry dishes.

DO NOT OVERCOOK VEGETABLES. THEY SHOULD BE TENDER AND CRISP.

Equally important, do not attempt to keep vegetables warm for more than a few minutes. If you cannot serve at once, it is better to remove them from the heat, set aside, and reheat later. Overcooking and keeping vegetables hot ruins the color, texture, and taste, as well as most of the nutritive qualities.

Note: Although vegetables will yield brighter colors when cooked with baking soda, their nutritional levels may be drastically reduced.

*AICR — *American Institute for Cancer Research*

# ARTICHOKES

Artichokes are available year round but peak season is March through May. Artichokes are a nutritional bonus: A good source of calcium, phosphorus, and iron, they are also rich in iodine, a hard-to-find nutrient. A little known artichoke fact is their potassium richness: A medium-sized artichoke contains about 210 milligrams of potassium, along with vitamins A, B, and C. Artichokes are also low in sodium and contain only about 0.2% fat.

The versatile artichoke makes a wonderful appetizer, main dish, or salad, and goes well with seafood.

*Purchase* — Choose artichokes that are bright green and have tightly packed leaves (or bracts). Buy small, medium, or large artichokes, since all are fully mature and ready to cook.

*Store* — Do not wash before storing. An artichoke will look and stay fresh up to 2 weeks in the refrigerator. Place in plastic bag to keep longer.

*Use* — Wash artichoke under running water, remove lower leaves, and trim the bottom of the stem so the artichoke can stand upright. If serving children, you may want to cut off the sharp tips of the leaves. To prevent discoloring, sprinkle with fresh lemon juice. To boil: Place artichokes in a large pan, with enough room to stand upright. Add a couple of Tablespoons of lemon juice and about 3 inches of water. Cover and bring to a boil, reduce heat and simmer 15-25 minutes, or until bottoms are fork tender.

Artichokes are slightly awkward to eat, especially if it is your first meeting. Start by breaking off each leaf with your fingers, dip bottom "broken off part" into desired sauce, then scrape the bottom of the leaf off between your teeth. Discard leaf. Provide a "discard" leaf plate. After you have eaten all the leaves, take a knife and scrape off the fuzzy choke in the center to get to the heart at the bottom. The heart has a nutty flavor.

A serving hint to make it easier on your family or guests: After cooking, pull out the purple-tipped prickly leaves in the center and scrape out the fuzzy choke with a spoon to reveal the heart.

74

## ASPARAGUS

Asparagus is a very popular member of the lily family. Peak season is March through June. Asparagus provides vitamins A and C, and potassium.

*Purchase* — Choose plump, firm stalks with compact tips and good green color. The cut end should not be woody or too dry.

*Store* — Keep in plastic bag up to 1 week in refrigerator, or slice off bottoms of stems and stand upright in an inch or 2 of water in the refrigerator. You can also wrap a damp cloth around the cut ends and place in refrigerator. Do not wash until ready to use. Eat as soon as possible for best flavor.

*Use* — To steam, use large pan and place asparagus upright with 2 inches of water and steam 10-15 minutes. Note: If you don't have an asparagus steamer, an old-fashioned coffee percolator makes a good substitute.

To bake, place in baking dish 1 layer thick, sprinkle with lemon juice, cover with foil and bake at 350° for 15-20 minutes. The asparagus will cook in its own juice.

Remember, too, that asparagus is absolutely delicious raw.

I prefer to peel the stems of the asparagus to be sure that the whole spear is edible.

## AVOCADO

Avocados are available year round. They are botanically fruits, but are more often served as vegetables. They provide vitamins A, B, C, E, and K, potassium, iron, magnesium, and are 60% water. Half an avocado has more potassium than a banana, is low in sodium, and has no cholesterol. Avocados have a creamy texture with a delicate nutlike flavor. Provides 250 calories per $3^1/_2$ ounces (100 grams) of pulp.

*Purchase* — Most avocados are sold firm and must soften before they are edible. Choose the unblemished ones and let ripen in a warm place (preferably on your kitchen counter) until soft to the touch, then refrigerate until ready to use.

*Use* — The versatile avocado can be used for more than

guacamole. It can be served with cheese and fruit, cut in half and stuffed with crab, tuna, or chicken (to name a few), or just served plain with lemon juice and your favorite crackers. Add to sandwiches, tacos, omelettes, salads, etc.

To avoid the brownish color that develops when the avocado's flesh is exposed to air, sprinkle with fresh lemon juice.

If avocado is prepared before it's time to be eaten, the stone should be left in the dish with the pulp; otherwise, it will turn black and appear unappetizing.

## BEETS

Beets are available year round, with peak season being June through October. They provide vitamins A and C, potassium, and other minerals. Beets are not given much credit even though they are very versatile. They can be eaten raw or used in salads, and are famous in borscht or as pickled beets. Beet greens are highly nutritious, providing vitamins A and C. The smaller the beet root, the more tender the greens. Try them. Beet tops are great in salads, or cooked in the same way as spinach.

*Purchase* — Choose beets that are firm, smooth, and without soft spots. Medium-sized beets have the best flavor. Beet tops should be dark green with red veins. If they look dry and brown, you'll know that the crown was not underground and will probably be tough as well.

*Store* — Cut off tops of beets, leaving about an inch of stem. Store beets in plastic bag in refrigerator. Will keep 1-3 weeks. Wash when ready to use. Store beet greens in plastic bag in refrigerator for up to one week.

*Use* — Cook beets in their skins, without tops, in a small amount of water until tender. Skins will slip off readily after cooking. Small beet roots cook in 30-45 minutes. If you prefer, you can peel before cooking.

# BELL PEPPERS

There are two groups of peppers: Sweet and mild, and hot and spicy. The bell pepper is the sweetest and largest and is available in green, red, yellow, and purple varieties. The brightly colored ones have merely been allowed to ripen longer, and they taste sweeter than the green ones. All varieties provide vitamins A, B, and C.

*Purchase* — Choose crisp, firm bell peppers without discoloration or soft spots.

*Store* — Refrigerate; will keep about 1 week.

*Use* — In stir-fry, or stuffed with meat, chicken or seafoods. Try raw with dips or in salads.

# BROCCOLI

Broccoli is a member of the cabbage family. It provides vitamins A and C, iron, calcium, phosphorus, and potassium. Available year round.

*Purchase* — Choose dark green heads, with buds that are tightly closed in compact clusters. Do not buy broccoli showing yellow flowers through the buds. It is old and will taste woody and musty. Stalks should be green without signs of drying along the sides.

*Store* — In refrigerator about 1 week.

*Use* — Broccoli has a great taste and is delicious in salads, stir-fry, vegetable casseroles, and soups. Wash, trim leaves and stem ends. If time allows, soak broccoli in cold water 5-10 minutes before cooking. Best when steamed — cover and steam 10-20 minutes, depending on size of head. Cook until crisp, but tender. Do not overcook. It should still be bright green after steaming.

# BRUSSELS SPROUTS

Peak season mid-August through April. Provide vitamins A and C, potassium, and iron. Brussels sprouts resemble miniature cabbages 1-2 inches in diameter, and have a robust nutlike flavor. They are a tradition with turkey at an English Christmas dinner.

*Purchase* — Look for small, firm, green Brussels sprouts. Avoid those with yellowing leaves. Older sprouts tend to be coarse in texture, with a strong flavor and odor, while smaller ones are tender and have a mild flavor.

*Store* — In plastic bag in refrigerator. Use within a few days for best flavor.

*Use* — Wash. Trim stems and remove any discolored leaves. Do not overcook. Sprouts should be slightly crunchy, not mushy. They are great steamed, served plain, or with favorite sauces, and can be baked, puréed, or added to soups and casseroles. To boil, place in rapidly boiling water, cover, and cook 10-15 minutes, depending on size, until tender.

## *CABBAGE*

Cabbage is over 90% water, is a good source of fiber, and has traces of protein, carbohydrate, and fat. Cabbage contains moderate amounts of vitamins A, B-complex, magnesium, calcium, and potassium, with less than 35 calories per cup. Available year round, 1 pound equals $2^1/_2$ cups of shredded or cooked cabbage.

**Danish Cabbage** — Danish cabbage includes varieties that mature late in the season and develop hard, tight, compact heads. Usually white in color with round or flat heads. Most suitable cabbage for winter storage.

**Green Cabbage (Domestic)** — Green cabbage is the most popular type, has flat or rounded heads with compact leaves, pale green in color. Often used to make sauerkraut.

**Red or Purple Cabbage** — Red or purple cabbage has slightly more vitamin C than green cabbage. Otherwise, it looks similar to green cabbage, but has reddish, purple, and white streaks on leaves.

**Savoy Cabbage** — Savoy cabbage is yellow-green in color and has loose, ruffled leaves with tall loose heads, somewhat resembling romaine lettuce in shape. Others have tight heads surrounded by huge open leaves. Savoy cabbages are more tender than domestic, with a milder flavor.

*Purchase* — Cabbages should be solid hard, heavy in relation to size, with crisp leaves. Avoid cabbages with insect damage, decay, yellowing leaves, or cracked heads. Examine the base of the cabbage. If some of the outer leaves are separated and held in place only by the folding of leaves over the head, do not buy — such heads may be overly strong in flavor and tough in texture.

*Store* — Keep tightly wrapped in plastic bag. Will keep about 2 weeks refrigerated. Do not remove outer leaves until ready to use as they help retain moisture. If already cut, rub lemon juice on the cut edges to minimize discoloration.

*Use* — Use in salads, sautéed, stir-fried, stuffed, or baked. Cooked cabbage goes well with other vegetables, meats, poultry, and fish. However, DO NOT OVERCOOK — it intensifies an unpleasant odor and greatly reduces the nutritional value. Cabbage should be added near the end of cooking time when added to soups, stews, or casseroles.

## CHINESE CABBAGE

There are several varieties of Chinese cabbage, all low in calories, easily digested, and high in vitamin C. The flavors range from sweet to bitter. The following varieties are easily found in local or Asian markets.

**Bok Choy** (often marketed as Pak Choy) — Resembles chard, with a thick white stem and wide, very dark green leaves. Stalks are crisp with a slight bitterness. Available year round. Eaten raw in salads, stir-fried, or added to soups. A nice complement for seafood or beef.

**Chinese Mustard** (sometimes called mustard cabbage, or big stem mustard) — Chinese mustards vary in appearance. They can be dark green, red, or variegated with green or red fuzzy leaves and contorted shapes. The smaller leaves have a bittersweet flavor, while the older leaves are stronger tasting. Usually used in stews, soups, stir-fried, or pickled. Wash, discard the tough stems, peel fibers from the midribs if necessary because of toughness.

**Flat Cabbage** — A member of the cabbage family, the leaves are dark green and spoonlike in shape and the head looks flattened. Found in specialty shops. Flat cabbage may be substituted for bok choy, but has a stronger flavor.

**Flowering White Cabbage** — Flowering white cabbage has thick stems and flowering shoots, often confused with Chinese broccoli. (Flowering white cabbage has lighter stems.) Can be used like any other green.

**Michili Cabbage** (also called celery cabbage or Chinese cabbage) — Some michili cabbages have pale blond leaves that tuck inward, while others have leaves that flare out from the top of the head. Has longer, slimmer leaves than nappa cabbage, with a stronger flavor.

**Nappa Cabbage** — Nappa cabbage is the most common Chinese cabbage in the U.S. Has pale green, firm, stout heads. Nappa cabbage has a delicious mild flavor. Used raw in salads, or cooked in soups, vegetable dishes, stir-fry, and stews.

**Pe-Tsai** (also called celery cabbage) — Pe-Tsai forms a conical or rectangular shape, with a compact head. Looks similar to romaine lettuce. Has a mild flavor and is best in stir-fry dishes.

*Store* — Thoroughly wash greens, drain well, and store in plastic bag in refrigerator for 1-2 weeks (may even be frozen).

## CARDOON

A close relative of the globe artichoke, but is eaten for its leafy stalks similar to celery. Cardoon only tastes vaguely like an artichoke. Nutritionally, cardoon provides vitamin B-complex and C, some protein, small amount of carbohydrate and fat. It is 90% water.

*Purchase* — Buy crisp bunches with fresh leaves.

*Store* — Store cardoon in a plastic bag in refrigerator, it will keep about a week.

*Use* — Cardoons are best tasting when blanched, otherwise they are too bitter. Before cooking, scrape the ribs of the fibers and prickles on the outside, cut into desired lengths. Cook 15-20 minutes depending on size. Serve with lemon juice, garlic butter, or cheese sauce. The tender leaves may also be eaten. Cook the same as spinach.

# CARROTS

The carrot, a member of the parsley family, is extremely high in vitamin A and selenium, along with other vitamins and minerals such as magnesium, phosphorus, and potassium. It also provides protein, carbohydrate, and fiber. A single carrot far exceeds the minimum daily adult requirement of vitamin A. Carrots are a great carry-along snack.

*Purchase* — Choose carrots with bright orange color that are not dried out, limp, or cracked. The slimmer ones are sweeter, and have a smaller core.

*Store* — Keep in refrigerator up to 2 weeks. Do not wash until ready to use.

*Use* — The carrot's uses are endless in juice, salads, steamed, baked, and creamed.

1 medium carrot = $2^1/_2$-3 ounces

1 pound sliced or diced carrots = $3^1/_2$-4 cups

# CAULIFLOWER

Cauliflower is available year round, and is a member of the cabbage family. Provides vitamins A and C, calcium, protein, carbohydrates, fiber, and iron. Cauliflower is easily distinguished from broccoli until you run into a green or purple cauliflower.

*Purchase* — Look for firm cauliflower, creamy white in color with no blemishes. The curd should be closely packed, not mealy or separated. Old cauliflower takes on a strong odor and flavor.

*Store* — Trim stem ends and any leaves. Store in plastic bag in refrigerator. Will keep for about a week. Do not wash until ready to use.

*Use* — You can cook cauliflower whole, but do not eat the woody base. When most of us think of cauliflower, we think of it covered with cheese sauce, but there are many other uses for it. Cauliflower tastes great raw in dips, relish trays, and salads, or steamed, creamed, and even pickled.

# CELERIAC

Celeriac is low in calories and is a good source of fiber. Has a turnip-shaped root with a rough brown skin. The small roots are less woody than the larger ones. Celeriac is not related to celery but is actually from the carrot family. It has a sweet celery-parsley flavor and a crunchy texture.

*Purchase* — Choose roots that are firm and heavy for their size. Fresh celeriac has a strong smell and a dirty appearance.

*Store* — Keep in plastic bag in refrigerator. Will keep about 1 week.

*Use* — May be peeled and eaten raw, or peeled and blanched in water with 2 Tablespoons of lemon juice added to get rid of a slightly bitter taste. Great eaten plain, in salads, soups, or combined with potatoes.

# CELERY

Celery is a member of the parsley family and has been known by cooks for thousands of years. Provides vitamins A and C, sodium, and potassium.

*Purchase* — Buy crisp bunches with fresh leaves.

*Store* — Refrigerate. Will last about a week or so in the refrigerator.

*Use* — Can be eaten raw, stuffed, in soups, stews, stir-fry, salads and, of course, in poultry stuffing. The leaves are a flavorful addition to soups and stews.

2 sliced stalks of celery stalks = $^3/_4$-1 cup

A welcome addition to a variety of dishes.

# CHAYOTE

Chayote is a member of the gourd family, is available year round, and provides protein and fiber. It is a tropical summer squash, shaped like a deeply ridged papaya, with 1 large seed and a bland taste and firm texture.

*Purchase* — Choose firm chayote with a nice pale green color and unblemished skin with no brown spots.

*Store* — In plastic bag in refrigerator. Will keep about 3 weeks.

*Use* — Wash. Cut in half, remove the seed, and peel. Chayote can be baked, steamed, or prepared like other squash. Good in soups or stews. Needs strong seasonings, because, like eggplant, it will absorb the seasonings.

## *CORN*

Corn's peak season is June through October. Corn provides vitamins A and C, protein, amino acids, minerals, and carbohydrates. It is absolutely at its best when you buy it from a local source and eat it the day it is picked. When not in season, frozen corn, whole or in kernel form, is usually very good.

*Purchase* — Buy ears with fresh green husks and golden but not dry silk threads. Look for firm, smallish kernels with no mold or decay at tip of cob.

*Store* — Use fresh corn the day you buy it or as soon as you can for best flavor. Keep refrigerated.

*Use* — Fresh corn can be eaten raw, or cooked in boiling water for 7 minutes. It is wonderful cooked in its husks on your barbecue coals. It is sweet, tender, and juicy. Corn can be used in a variety of recipes, from soups to breads to salads.

## *CUCUMBER*

Do not peel. Cucumbers are about 96% water and most of the vitamins they have are contained in the skin. Cucumbers are a member of the gourd family and have a cool, refreshing taste, available year round.

*Purchase* — Choose firm, slender, medium-sized cucumbers with bright green skin. Avoid the large, fat, older ones, which are mostly seeds and can be dry and bitter.

*Store* — Wash well. Store in refrigerator up to 1 week. Do not cut until ready to use.

*Use* — Cucumbers are excellent thinly sliced on a sandwich, in salads, soups, cut into sticks for dips, and, of course, are indispensable as pickles. Also, cucumbers are a great facial cleanser and eye relaxer.

There are two categories of cucumbers — slicing and pickling.

**Slicing** — Lemon, English, and Green Market cucumbers.

**Pickling** — Dill, Cornichons, and West Indian Gherkin cucumbers.

## EGGPLANT

Western eggplant belongs to the solanaceous family, and is related to potatoes, tomatoes, and peppers. Color ranges from creamy white to yellow, brown, purple, and even black. It has long, slender, or round, egg-shaped fruit. Cooked eggplant is 94% water and provides minimal amounts of vitamins and minerals. Peak season is July through August.

*Purchase* — Look for eggplant with taut, unwrinkled, shiny skin. Old eggplants develop bitter skins and tough seeds.

*Store* — Keeps in refrigerator up to 1 week.

*Use* — Eggplant is extremely versatile; being spongy and bland, it absorbs whatever seasonings you add to it. Combines well with foods such as cheeses, tomatoes, meats, and is well known in the Greek dish moussaka.

## FENNEL

A member of the parsley family, fennel looks similar to celery with very feathery leaves. The whole plant has a sweet anise (licorice) flavor. Fennel provides vitamin A, calcium, and potassium. A winter vegetable available October through May.

*Purchase* — Choose crisp, firm, compact bulbs with fresh-looking leaves.

*Store* — Refrigerate in a plastic bag. Will keep 4-5 days. Do not separate stalks. Wash when ready to use.

*Use* — Wash. Trim the bottom and top. Remove outer pieces if they are bruised. Fennel can be eaten raw, steamed, or baked. Great in Italian dishes, soups, fish dishes, or alone.

Note: There are two types of fennel — the heading type (the herb) and the bulbous type (the vegetable).

## *HORSERADISH*

Peak seasons are April through May, and October through early December. A member of the cabbage family, horseradish provides vitamin C. It is believed that the Germans were the first to use horseradish as a condiment rather than a medicine. It was sliced thin and mixed with vinegar, to be eaten with meat or fish. Today, horseradish with vinegar is a popular condiment for prime rib, corned beef hash, baked potatoes, and in seafood and other sauces.

*Purchase* — Look for smooth, unblemished roots, 5-12 inches long.

*Store* — Fresh horseradish will keep about 1 month, and may also be frozen.

*Use* — When using fresh horseradish, peel and grate the root. Be ready . . . it is worse than peeling onions! Or buy prepared horseradish!

Check Uncle Al's recipe on page 138.

## *JERUSALEM ARTICHOKE*

Jerusalem artichokes (also called sun chokes) are a good source of iron, and contain vitamins A and B-complex, potassium, and calcium. They have a sweet nutty flavor and a crunchy texture. Available year round. Introduce them slowly into your diet. They sometimes cause flatulence after eating a number of them.

*Purchase* — Jerusalem artichokes come in irregular shapes. Select the smoothest ones, 2-6 inches long, and firm to the touch.

*Store* — Keep in plastic bag in refrigerator. Will keep about 1 week.

*Use* — Wash, peel, and eat raw in salads or as crudités. They can also be steamed, baked, or broiled. Delicious puréed and added to mashed potatoes, sautéed, and in stews. You can even use them in a pie.

Note: Do not cook in an aluminum pan, or tubers will turn black. A nutritious flour can be made by grinding dried Jerusalem artichokes.

## JICAMA

Jicama (hee´-ka-ma) is a tuber of the morning glory family. It has a thick brown skin and is shaped like a turnip. Jicama is sweet, juicy, and very crunchy, like water chestnuts.

*Purchase* — Choose firm jicama with no blemishes.

*Store* — Will keep in refrigerator for up to 1 week. Do not cut until ready to use or it will dry out.

*Use* — Jicama can be eaten raw or cooked. Peel and dice to add crunch to a salad, or add to stir-fry.

## KOHLRABI

Kohlrabi (kohl-ra´-bi) provides vitamin C, potassium, calcium, and magnesium. Peak season is June through July.

Kohl (German for cabbage) and rabi (German for turnip) are clues to its taste and texture. Kohlrabi is a member of the cabbage family, but has a swollen stem that resembles a turnip. Depending on the variety, the skin may be purple, green, or light green. The flesh is white, with a crunchy texture and a sweet cabbage flavor. Turnips and kohlrabi are interchangeable in most recipes.

*Purchase* — Bulbs can grow as big as grapefruits, but the larger ones tend to be woody in texture. Kohlrabi is best when about the size of an orange. If the skin is tough, peel it off. If you find kohlrabi with leaves still attached, remember that they are edible, too.

*Store* — Cut off leaves and trim root, wash in cold water, pat dry. Store in plastic bag in refrigerator for up to a week.

*Use* — Can be eaten raw, steamed, or cooked in broth.

To crisp for salad — soak in ice water for 15 minutes before using.

## LEEK

Leeks provide vitamin C, calcium, and phosphorus, and are a good source of potassium. Leeks are members of the onion family, with a stalk rather than a bulb. They look like overgrown scallions, very pale in color, with tightly rolled, flat, and straplike leaves. They tend to turn mushy quickly, so do not overcook.

*Purchase* — Buy leeks that are white at the base, with tightly rolled, pale green leaves. The smaller ones are more tender.

*Store* — Cut off roots and the last inch or so of leaves. Store leeks in plastic bag in refrigerator. Be sure to wash well before using, since soil tends to get into layers of the leaves.

*Use* — Leeks can be used in almost any dish you desire — omelettes, soups, stir-fry, salads, etc.

## LOTUS ROOT

Lotus root has a bland flavor but is valued for its crunchy texture and irregular design. It is a member of the lily family, and provides potassium, with traces of calcium, magnesium, phosphorus, and vitamin C. Great used in salads and stir-fry. Choose firm root without any signs of mold or soft spots. Wash and peel, slice crosswise.

## MUSHROOMS

Mushrooms provide vitamin B, amino acids, iron, selenium, and copper. They are available year round. Mushrooms are fungi that live in darkness, feeding off other organic matter.

*Purchase* — When buying white mushrooms look for tan/white ones with closed caps that do not show undergills. Mushrooms are highly perishable. Avoid any that are chipped or have black spots. It is advisable to buy mushrooms in bulk rather than pre-packaged, so that you can hand pick each one.

$^1/_2$ pound of sliced fresh mushrooms = about $2^1/_2$ cups

$^1/_2$ pound of diced fresh mushrooms = about 2 cups

*Store* — Keep mushrooms in a paper bag in the refrigerator. Will keep about a week. Use plastic bag only if you plan on using mushrooms right away, or they will turn soggy. Wash gently under running water or wipe with a damp cloth before using.

*Use* — Can be added to almost any recipe, sliced raw in salads, stuffed, steamed, or sautéed — their uses are endless.

## ENOKITAKE MUSHROOMS *(e´-no-key-tah-kay´)*

Also called Enoki-dake or Enoki, Enokitake mushrooms provide vitamins B and C, potassium, iron, and phosphorus, and are available year round. Look for tiny caps on thin stems, connected in a cluster at the base. Raw, Enokitake mushrooms have a crisp, mild taste.

*Purchase* — Enokitake are sold in clusters wrapped in plastic, about 3½ ounces. Check stems to make sure they are not turning brown or wilted. Should be white with no blemishes.

*Store* — Refrigerate. Will keep about a week.

*Use* — Try in salads or use in soups and stir-fry dishes. They are very delicate and will toughen if overcooked, so add last. Available at your supermarket or Japanese market.

## SHIITAKE MUSHROOMS *(she-tah´-kay)*

Shiitake mushrooms are also called Oriental black mushrooms, or golden oak mushrooms. They provide vitamin B, protein, calcium, and phosphorus. Until recently these mushrooms were only available in dried form. Soak the dried variety in warm water until they become puffy; rinse and use. Japanese cooks find shiitake mushrooms indispensable.

*Purchase* — Some cooks say the best shiitake mushrooms have a network of creamy colored fissures on the caps. Choose firm and dry mushrooms, make sure they are moist without dark spots showing rot. They should have a woody odor but not overly strong.

*Store* — In refrigerator (damp cloth helps hold in moisture). Will keep about 1½-2 weeks.

*Use* — Their pungent flavor lends great taste to any recipe, and they are a delicious treat.

# OKRA

Okra provides vitamins A and C, calcium, and potassium, and very few calories. Peak season is July through October. Okra is actually the immature seed pod of the hibiscus plant, finger-shaped and lightly covered with fine hairs. The pods resemble green chili peppers. Is a member of the mallow family, and a warm weather plant. Cooked okra has a slippery texture.

**Chinese Okra** — Huge, with crisp skin and squash-like flavor. Choose gourds about 1 foot long with firm, ridged skin and a fresh dark green color. Resembles a giant version of okra.

*Purchase* — Choose small, crisp, blemish-free pods, 1-4 inches long. Okra should snap easily when broken.

*Store* — Keep in refrigerator in plastic bag. Both types will keep about 1 week. Use before the pods become limp or discolored.

*Use* — Wash when ready to use, trim stem ends. Great pickled, fried, or stewed. In stews, okra acts as a thickener. The Chinese kind is good in stir-fry cooking. In the south, okra is considered an essential ingredient in gumbos or Creole dishes. My Texan friend Christine likes it pickled.

Cut okra at the last moment before cooking, otherwise it releases its mucilage.

# ONION

Dry onion bulbs come in many shapes, sizes, and colors — yellow, brown, purple, or white, elongated or round. Bermuda onions are mild, and Walla Walla onions are sweet. Onions provide protein, calcium, phosphorus, iron, and vitamins B and C. Green onions also have vitamin A, magnesium, and potassium, with traces of other vitamins and minerals.

*Purchase* — Select hard, firm bulbs with clean skin. Avoid bulbs that are sprouting or damp.

*Store* — Keep in a dry, cool location. Whole onions can be kept up to 1 month. I store my onions in the pantry hanging in a pair of pantyhose. Drop onion in, tie a knot, drop in another onion, tie knot, etc. When you need an onion, just cut off from the bottom. This method cuts down on mold and spoilage.

*Use* — In almost anything.

1 medium onion = 2½-3 ounces

1 pound sliced or diced onions equals 3½-4 cups

## GREEN ONIONS

Green onions are sometimes called scallions, and have a milder flavor than dry onions. Green onions are young, small-bulbed onions, used mostly for their leaves.

*Purchase* — Buy green onions with crisp, green, unblemished leaves.

*Store* — About 1 week in refrigerator.

*Use* — They are delicious served in salads, relish trays, stir-fry, and soups, to name a few.

## SHALLOTS

Shallots are a cross between garlic and onion, shaped somewhat like a garlic bulb with tissue-wrapped cloves, but with a taste like a delicate onion.

1 medium shallot equals 1 Tablespoon when minced (or ½ ounce).

*Purchase* — Buy plump, firm bulbs. Avoid soft, shriveled ones.

*Store* — Will keep about 1 month in ventilated place.

## PEARL ONIONS

Small white bulbs, used in pickling, boiling, marinating, or in cocktails. Available year round. Bulbs should be firm.

## CHIVES

Small, thin, spiky tops with essentially no bulbs. Used as an herb, fresh or dried.

# GARLIC

Garlic is a member of the onion family, and each garlic bulb consists of 8-20 cloves attached to a root-base. Each individual clove is covered with a purplish or white skin, surrounded by a white papery covering. (A clove of garlic is one section.) There is a larger variety of garlic called elephant or tahiti garlic. This has 5-6 large cloves per bulb, is milder than regular garlic, and may be used as liberally as shallots, onions, or leeks. Garlic provides no outstanding amounts of vitamins or minerals, but preliminary medical research indicates garlic's power to lower blood cholesterol levels. There is speculation that garlic may have antibiotic properties and some protective value against heart disease, stroke, cancer, and diabetes. Garlic enhances the flavor of food without adding a lot of extra calories.

*Purchase* — Choose garlic that is firm and heavy to the touch, with no soft spots. Avoid shriveled, stained or sprouting garlic.

*Store* — If properly stored, garlic will keep 6 months (in warm weather) to a year in cooler weather. Refrigeration is not recommended because too much humidity will cause garlic to mildew.

2-3 medium cloves equals 1 teaspoon fresh crushed or puréed garlic.

1-2 medium cloves equals 1 teaspoon minced garlic.

1 medium clove of fresh garlic equals 1/8 teaspoon.

To remove the odor of garlic from your hands, rinse hands in cold water, rub with table salt, rinse again in cold water, then wash hands with soap and water. Repeat if necessary.

*Use* — Garlic enhances any dish: Chicken, seafood, salads, dressings, soups. Try using garlic instead of salt or extra fat. Remember to peel clove unless otherwise directed.

*Blanching garlic* — Blanching develops a delicious flavor. In a saucepan, bring about 1 quart of water to a boil. Separate a head of garlic, add unpeeled cloves to boiling water, boil about 30 seconds. Drain, peel garlic cloves, place in a saucepan of cold water, bring to a boil again, then drain.

Alternate method: Break apart garlic head, drop unpeeled cloves into saucepan with water to cover, boil uncovered until cloves are tender (about 3 minutes for small cloves to 10 minutes for large cloves), drain, and cool. When cool enough to handle, pinch tips between thumb and forefingers to squeeze garlic skins off. Baking produces a mild, sweet, nutty flavor.

## PARSNIPS

Parsnips provide carbohydrates, vitamins A and C, and potassium. Peak season is October through January. Parsnips resemble carrots. The root is tasty and rather sweet, but is tougher than carrots, with a texture similar to that of a sweet potato.

*Purchase* — Select smooth parsnips, firm to the touch, with a creamy white color. Avoid the larger ones which are usually fibrous with a woody core. Stay away from soft or flabby ones also.

*Store* — Refrigerate. Will keep about a month.

*Use* — Scrub, trim both ends. Great in soups and stews, shredded raw in salads, or sautéed in olive oil. Parsnips can be substituted for rutabagas and sweet potatoes.

## PEAS

Peas provide protein, vitamins A, B and C, iron, amino acids, and magnesium. Peak season is March through May. Peas are best when fresh. They are worth the extra time spent in shelling.

*Purchase* — Pick small shiny green pods. The big faded pods will taste starchy and old.

*Store* — Refrigerate, unshelled, in plastic bag and eat as soon as possible.

*Use* — Steamed as a side dish, in salads, creamed, and in stir-fry dishes.

## SNOWPEAS

Snowpeas, also called sugar peas or Chinese pea pods, provide vitamins A and C, minerals, and are a good source of protein. Snowpeas have crisp, flat pods and almost invisible seeds.

*Purchase* — Look for crisp, flat pods with no bulging peas. Larger peas are a sign of age.

*Store* — In refrigerator in a plastic bag to retain moisture. Use within a few days.

*Use* — Serve whole. Snap off the ends and string them (like green beans). Sweet, crisp, raw peas are good as dippers, and are delicious parboiled with olive oil and herbs added. Of course, they are excellent in stir-fry dishes, or with meat and chicken dishes. Keep cooking time to a minimum to retain texture, color and flavor. Add to recipe last if rest of ingredients call for longer cooking time.

## POTATOES

Potatoes are available year round, and provide vitamins B, B2 and C, iron, carbohydrates, potassium, calcium, and phosphorus. They are a very good diet food if you do not load them up with sour cream, butter, and bacon. A medium-sized potato contains only about 125 calories, a large one about 200 calories.

*Purchase* — Look for potatoes that are blemish-free with no greenish color or sprouting eyes.

*Store* — Do not refrigerate. Store in a dry, cool place. Will keep about 3 weeks.

1 medium potato = $3^1/_2$-4 ounces

1 pound of sliced or diced potatoes yields $3^1/_2$-4 cups

1 pound unpeeled raw potatoes = about 2 cups mashed potatoes

*Use* — Potatoes are very versatile, and can be used as a side dish or main dish, in soups, stews, dumplings, even potato pizza on page 345.

## RADISH

The radish is a member of the cabbage family, provides vitamin C, and is available year round. Radishes come in all shapes, sizes, and colors, including black. Cherry-sized red radishes are the most common variety sold.

*Purchase* — Look for crisp, well-formed, smooth radishes with fresh green leaves. Avoid yellowed, wilted or cracked radishes.

*Store* — To clean, remove tops, wash, and refrigerate about 1 week; or trim top and bottom of radish and set into a bowl of cold water, keep in refrigerator.

*Use* — Radishes can be cooked like turnips, but taste best raw in salads or relish trays.

**Daikon Radish** — An Oriental radish, daikon is a huge, white radish that is commonly used in Oriental dishes. They are milder than the common garden radish, and produce white roots 2-4 inches in diameter, and 6-20 inches long. Use in stir-fry, salads, pickled, or boil as other vegetables.

# RUTABAGA

The rutabaga was created less than 200 years ago, and is a cross between a turnip and a cabbage. It has yellow flesh that is firmer than a turnip, and purple-yellow skin. Provides protein, potassium, folacin, calcium, and phosphorus. Available all year, but freshest in the fall and winter.

*Purchase* — Select small to medium sizes, as the large ones may be woody or fibrous. Roots should be firm, not soft.

*Store* — Will keep about a week in the refrigerator.

*Use* — Wash, remove leaves, and trim ends. Peel and steam, or boil until tender and serve with margarine and cheese, or add to stews. Some cooks prefer to peel after cooking.

# SQUASH

Squash come in so many sizes, shapes, and colors that a simple description is difficult. Squash are most commonly grouped as either summer squash (the soft-skinned variety) or winter squash (the hard-skinned variety).

## SUMMER SQUASH

These varieties are mostly water, but provide a fair amount of vitamins A and C, potassium, and calcium. They are available year round. Summer squash are eaten when immature, with underdeveloped seeds and thin skins. As a rule, the larger summer squash have less flavor and tougher texture. Choose firm, tender squash, with no soft or brown spots. Use as soon as possible. They will keep about 1 week refrigerated. Wash, trim stem end, but do not peel. Use raw in salads, stir-fried with other vegetables, sautéed, with pasta, in soups, stews, baked, or steamed.

**Caserta and Coczelle** — Dark green skin like a zucchini, except caserta has light green stripes, and coczelle has yellow stripes. Best when 6-8 inches long.

**Crookneck** — Crookneck has a bulbous base and a narrow, curving neck (although some strains have straight necks). They have yellow skin, with a bumpy, gourd-like appearance, and yellow flesh. Best when 8-10 inches in length, but they can grow much larger.

**Pattypan** (Scalloped) — Also called bush scallop or custard marrow. Pale green skin, turning white as it gets larger. There is also a yellow variety. Pattypan is round with scalloped edges, and a slightly bumpy skin. Choose squash 2-4 inches in diameter.

**Scallopini** — Scallopini is a cross between pattypan and zucchini, shaped like a pattypan squash, but colored like a zucchini. Use as you would pattypan or zucchini in recipes.

**Zucchini** — Although zucchini can grow to the size of a baseball bat, they are best eaten when 4-8 inches long. Zucchini are very versatile: Raw as crudités or in salads, stuffed, baked, sautéed, added to soups, stews, breads, even jams. Provides vitamin C, and can be eaten skin, seeds, and all. Colors range from white and pale gray to dark green, to yellow.

## WINTER SQUASH

These varieties are a rich source of vitamin A and potassium, with notable amounts of vitamin C, calcium, and fiber. They also contain some protein and carbohydrate. Available year round, but most plentiful fall through winter. Choose squash that's heavy for its size, with a hard, tough rind. Avoid squash with moldy or soft spots, punctures, or decaying cracks. A tender rind indicates immaturity. Winter squash will keep about a month at room temperature. For winter storage, cure squash by holding at 85° for 10 days, and then store in a cool, dry place. It will keep about 3 months. Do not refrigerate winter squash — the chill will diminish the flavor. Winter squash are delicious baked, steamed, puréed, or peeled, cubed, and added to soups or stews. Roast the seeds in a slow oven for a great snack.

**Acorn** — Acorn squash has a golden, fibrous texture and a sweet flavor. The skin is dark green with deep ridges, but changes to orange as it matures. Choose squash 6-8 inches long and about 4 inches in diameter. Great baked, sautéed, puréed, or added to soups. To bake, cut in half, remove seeds, bake at 350° for 45 minutes (cover halves with foil so they don't dry out), or microwave (full power) for 10-12 minutes for 2 halves.

**Asian** — A generic term for squash popular in Asia, often flat, or shaped like a football, weighing up to 15 pounds. Flesh is yellow/orange, and flavor is bland.

**Banana** — A large, elongated squash, up to 2 feet long. Skin color turns from green to yellow/pink, with orange flesh. Flavor is sweet and texture is creamy. Squash is ready to cook whole. Bake a 1-1½ pound squash in a conventional oven for 1 hour, or microwave for 10-12 minutes.

**Buttercup** — Also called turban because of the turban-shaped blossom end. Buttercup squash is usually about 8 inches across the top and 5 inches long. Has dark green skin, with a green/blue and orange/green turban. The flesh is sweet and bright orange.

**Butternut** — This squash is rather bell-shaped, and its hard skin is a light brown/orange in color. The flesh has a sweet, nutty flavor and is orange/yellow in color. To bake, cut in half, remove seeds, and bake at 350° for 1 hour, or microwave (full power) for 12-15 minutes for 2 halves.

**Chinese** — Has a sweet, creamy texture, and dark gold flesh. Average weight is about 2 pounds. To bake, cut in half, remove seeds, bake at 350° for 1 hour, or microwave (full power) 10-14 minutes for 2 halves.

**Delicata** — This squash is shaped somewhat like a large cucumber. Best when the skin is yellow with orange stripes. The flavor is very sweet, with a creamy texture. To bake, cut lengthwise, remove seeds, bake at 350° for 45 minutes, or microwave (full power) 8-12 minutes for 2 halves.

**Hubbard** — A large winter squash, its color varies from blue or gray-green, to dark green or red/orange. Skin is hard, with a pebbly, warted surface. These squash can weigh up to 30 pounds and have a nutty flavor and creamy texture. For approximately $1\frac{1}{2}$-pound squash, cut in half, remove seeds, bake at 350° for about 1 hour, or microwave (full power) 10-12 minutes.

**Kabacha** — This Japanese squash has a very sweet, nutty flavor and creamy texture, with light orange flesh. Size varies from 3-6 pounds. To bake, cut in half, remove seeds, bake at 350° for 1 hour or microwave (full power) 10-15 minutes.

**Spaghetti** — Spaghetti squash is unusual: Its flesh is composed of long threads that resemble spaghetti. The flavor is very bland and goes well with your favorite sauces. Its shape is round or elongated, and color is bright yellow. A 3-pound squash serves 4 people. Bake at 350°, whole or cut in half, for 45 minutes. Scrape spaghetti-like strands into serving bowl.

**Sweet Dumpling** (classified as an Asian squash) — This is an extremely tasty squash, 4 inches or more in diameter, with flavor most intense when skin is at yellow stage. To bake, cut in half, remove seeds, bake at 350° for 45 minutes, or microwave (full power) 8-10 minutes per squash.

**Tahitian** — Has a bulbous bottom and slightly curved neck. Seeds are located in the bottom of the cavity. Choose when skin is pale orange color. Flesh is also orange. May be eaten immature, when skin is green with yellow stripes and flesh is white.

**Warren Turban** — A larger variation of the buttercup squash, usually 8-10 inches long, and 12-15 inches across. They have a bright red/orange skin (sometimes striped) with a light blue turban. Flavor is very bland and goes well with favorite sauces.

**Pumpkin** — Pumpkins come in sizes up to 100 pounds. Skins are deep orange, or white in color, with yellow-orange flesh. A 5-pound pumpkin will yield $4\frac{1}{2}$ cups cooked and mashed pulp. A whole, uncut pumpkin will keep for 4-6 weeks if kept below 50°. If carved for Halloween, however, pumpkin should be used within 24 hours of carving. All scorched areas should be scraped off before cooking or the flavor of the pulp will be affected. If pumpkin is moldy it should be discarded. The idea of cutting off the mold and eating the remainder of the pulp is a dangerous one. The visible mold is only the bloom; the roots of the mold can spread throughout the pulp. Cooking and freezing are not reliable ways of eliminating mold.

Cooked, mashed, and frozen, pumpkin purée can be used in cakes, bread, pies, and cookies. Pumpkin seeds make a tasty and nutritious snack alone or mixed into your favorite granola, stuffings, or even tossed in a salad. These seeds are high in vitamins A and B, and contain traces of several minerals. Two Tablespoons of pumpkin seeds contain about 100 calories and 5 grams of protein. To prepare seeds for roasting, wash and remove any clinging pulp. Drain well, place on a cookie sheet and roast in oven at 250° for about 1-1½ hours or until golden brown. Mix seeds every 15 minutes. My dad likes to soak them overnight in salted water before roasting.

## SWEET POTATOES

Sweet potatoes, contrary to popular belief, are not related to white potatoes. White potatoes are tubers, while sweet potatoes are swollen roots. Sweet potatoes are high in vitamin A, and also contain vitamins B and C, iron, and phosphorus. The skins are a good source of fiber. Peak season is July through October. The most common variety of sweet potato has a bright orange-colored flesh, but there is another type which is drier and has paler colored, pinkish flesh.

*Purchase* — Choose sweet potatoes that are firm and blemish-free.

*Store* — Keep in a cool, dry place. Do not store in plastic or in the refrigerator.

*Use* — Sweet potatoes are extremely versatile: The small ones are perfect for baking and the larger ones can be stuffed, steamed, or puréed for pies or cookies. This is a vegetable that is fun to experiment with. Try honey and cinnamon in a baked sweet potato, for a real treat.

## TOMATILLO *(toe-ma´-tea-yo)*

Also called green tomato and husk tomato. The tomatillo has a lemony, acidic flavor. It is not from the same species as regular tomatoes, but belongs to the nightshade family, and is about the size of a cherry tomato. If not in your market, try the specialty shops. Tomatillos provide vitamin C. Peak season is September through November.

*Purchase* — Choose deep green color with tan husks. When fully ripe, tomatillos are often slightly purple in color, with a parchment-like husk.

*Store* — Keep in refrigerator in an airtight container; will keep about 10 days.

*Use* — Remove husks and wash, use whole. Seeding and peeling are not necessary. Tomatillo is a basic ingredient in salsa verde. Use raw in salads, or sautéed — great in ceviche, with chicken or in stews.

If cooking ahead of time for the next day, tomatillos should be blanched about 2 minutes in boiling water to avoid discoloration. They discolor after 6-8 hours.

## TOMATO

Tomatoes provide vitamins A and C, potassium, and iron. Available May through October. They range in size from baby cherry tomatoes to giant beefsteaks, and are best when vine-ripened.

*Purchase* — Choose tomatoes with the deepest red color. If tomato is still green, place in paper bag; this helps emit ethylene gas which ripens it. Do not refrigerate tomatoes unless overripe.

*Use* — Uses are endless, great in almost any dish.

## TURNIP

Turnips are members of the cabbage family. They provide vitamins A and C, and are available year round. Early turnips are small and tender, sometimes sold with the edible greens still on. The most common variety of turnip is round and white in color with a purplish crown. Has a faint peppery taste. Do not confuse with the yellow or orange rutabaga. The turnip has white flesh and is softer than a rutabaga.

*Purchase* — The best are heavy in relation to size and firm to the touch. Soft turnips are likely to be tough after cooking.

*Store* — Cut off tops, leaving about 1 inch of stem on root. The tops will keep a few days. Refrigerate. Turnips will keep about 3 weeks. Wash when ready to use.

*Use* — Use in soups or stews, steamed, puréed, or stir-fried.

**Turnip Tops** — Are the flowering tops of the turnip. Cook in the same manner as broccoli, then sauté in garlic and lemon juice.

# GREENS

Greens are the edible leaves of various plants. Leafy green vegetables are among the most nutritious and easiest to prepare. Some of these include mustard greens, beet greens, chard, Chinese cabbage, collard greens, dandelion greens, endive, kale, lettuce, parsley, radicchio, romaine, watercress, and spinach. These contain all or much of the adult daily requirements of vitamins A and C, as well as significant amounts of iron, calcium, riboflavin, niacin, and fiber. A $1/2$ cup serving of kale, for example, contains 90% of the daily adult vitamin A requirement and 85% of the daily adult vitamin C requirement, all for only 22 calories!

It is easy to get into a rut and keep choosing the same salad greens. For many of us, that may be iceberg lettuce only. It may be time to explore the leafy greens and discover or rediscover some of the delicious possibilities available to you.

Aside from providing the nutrition mentioned, they also provide a variety of flavors and textures. Greens are great in salads, sauces, and stir-fry, or steamed and served as a side dish. Greens are best when fresh, tender, and brightly colored. Avoid leaves that show insect damage, dry yellow color, excessive dirt, or a wilted appearance. Coarse stems may indicate over-maturity. I have listed a variety of greens and a brief description of each to help you choose a variety for your dinner table.

## ARUGULA

Also called Rocket, Roquette or Rucolo, is a member of the mustard family, with small, slender, notched, dark green leaves and a slightly bitter, peppery flavor. Use sparingly in mixed greens. Choose fairly smooth leaves. A furry underside is a sign of toughness.

**Wall Rocket** — Do not use alone, because of its sharp flavor. Use sparingly as a flavoring.

**Sea Rocket** — Use the youngest and tenderest shoots; like wall rocket use only as a flavoring.

## BEET GREENS

Highly nutritious and packed with vitamins A and C. The smaller the root, the more tender the greens. Great in salads or cooked like spinach.

## BUTTER or BOSTON LETTUCE

Small ruffled heads with delicate green leaves, and a mild flavor. Sometimes confused with bibb lettuce.

## CHARD (Swiss Chard)

Has broad green leaves that may be smooth or crinkled, and a delicate, tart flavor. It is actually a type of beet that does not develop a big red root. Tastes similar to spinach, and cooks in the same manner. When purchasing, look for plump stalks with tender leaves. Wash well, drain, discard bad leaves, and store in plastic bag in refrigerator. Will keep 1-2 weeks. Use in salads, soups, stir-fry, or substitute for spinach in most recipes.

## CHICORY

A family of strong-flavored greens that includes Belgian Endive, Grumolo, and Radicchios.

**Belgian** — Provides vitamins B1, B2, and C. Small spear-shaped heads. Choose crisp, tightly closed leaves that are creamy white with yellowish-green tips. Avoid any with blemishes. Refrigerate in plastic and use within 2-4 days. Serve raw in salads or braised. Although expensive, only a few leaves are needed to give a zesty lift.

**Grumolo** — Is a broad-leafed chicory, in a rounded bouquet, with a bitter taste.

**Radicchio** — There are three types: *Verona*, short leaves and rounded heart; *Red Treviso* with long and lanceolated leaves, with a more tapered heart; and *Castelfranco*, variegated chicory, green speckled leaves with red streaks with a round heart. Castelfranco is always eaten cooked.

**Wild Chicory** — The two best known bitter roots are *Bitter Chicory Root* and *Black Salsify*. Both are swollen roots, bitter but full of flavor. To use: Roots should be boiled and seasoned with lemon juice, or sautéed. Available year round, high in vitamins A and C, it is actually a wild Italian chicory. Red-leafed "green" grows in small, tight heads that look like small red cabbages — has a bitter flavor. Usually used as an accent rather than a main salad ingredient. Look for firm to hard heads, with deep purple-red leaves and white midribs. Refrigerate in plastic bag, will keep nearly a month.

## CHINESE CABBAGE

Has thick, broad, tender leaves with heavy midribs. Found in either loose or tight heads. To store: Trim roots, wash thoroughly, drain well, and store in plastic bag in refrigerator for 1-2 weeks (may be frozen). Good in salads, stir-fry, steamed, may even be used for cabbage rolls.

## CIMA DI RAPA

Also called broccoli de rabe, turnip tops, cima di rabe, raab, or rappini. A member of the cabbage family, cima di rapa is bitter or sweet, yellow or green, soft or crunchy. Available September through May. Look for a few fresh yellow flowers on the green florets, dark green leaves, and a strong stalk. Avoid those with wilted leaves or droopy florets. Wash, trim stem edges, discard large leaves and tough stalk ends. Available in Italian markets and specialty shops. Must be cooked slowly or it will acquire a bitter taste. Cook for 5 minutes. Also good eaten raw.

## COLLARDS

Sometimes called black cabbage. A member of the cabbage family, with smooth, dark green leaves that do not form heads. Good cooked, or raw in salads. Collards go especially well with ham and are similar to kale in texture and flavor. To store, wash thoroughly in cold water, drain well, remove damaged leaves, and keep in plastic bag for up to 1 week in refrigerator.

## CRESSES

There are several kinds of cresses. The following are the most widely available:

**Common Cress** — Also known as upland cress, winter cress, or pepper cress. It is available year round, although very hard to find in the markets. Its leaves resemble those of a small radish. Flavor is peppery and somewhat hot, the strongest of the cresses. Wash and trim stem ends.

**Garden Cress** — Like parsley, it can be used as an herb or a vegetable. Great in salads or on sandwiches. The smaller the leaves the better. There are both curly and flat-leafed varieties. Wash and trim stem ends.

**Watercress** — A member of the mustard family, its peak season is May through July. High in vitamins A and C, calcium, and iron, watercress is one of the oldest edible plants known to man. Has small, round, dark green leaves, with an aromatic, pleasantly sharp flavor. Often used as a garnish, excellent in salads, sauces, and soups. Choose fresh green bunches. Refrigerate and use as soon as possible. Highly perishable. Wash and then soak watercress for 10 minutes with a couple Tablespoons of white vinegar. This helps remove clinging insects.

**Bitter Cress** — Like watercress, it can be eaten alone or in salads to enhance the flavor of mixed greens with its pleasantly sharp flavor.

## CURLY ENDIVE

Provides vitamin A and iron. Has large rosettes of toothed, curled or wavy leaves. Use in salads or as a lettuce substitute. Available year round. Adds a distinct flavor. Wash thoroughly, drain, and refrigerate in plastic bag for up to 1 week.

# DANDELION GREENS

A special salad green in some parts of the world, especially in Europe. In spring, the leaves of the wild greens are mild, but develop a rather bitter flavor as they become larger. Some varieties are grown commercially in the U.S. and are bred to taste milder and grow larger than the wild plants. The nutritive value is similar to that of the various chicories. Very low in protein and carbohydrates, and no fat.

# ESCAROLE

Has long, flat leaves with pale yellow heart, and a tangy flavor. Look for tender crisp leaves with no signs of wilting.

# KALE

The young plants are the best. Peak season is December through April. A member of the cabbage family, the leaves are curly with fluted edges. Kale has a strong, peppery flavor, does not form a head, and is sometimes confused with collard greens. Wash in cold water and drain well. Remove damaged leaves. Store in plastic bag in refrigerator up to 1½-2 weeks. Kale can be used in salads, stir-fry, soups, and can even be stuffed.

**Chinese Kale** — Tastes a little like broccoli. Can be used in stir-fry, or prepared like broccoli.

# LETTUCE

**Leaf** — The ruffled leaves and mild-flavored lettuce that does not form a head. Includes red leaf lettuce with purplish edges and green leaf lettuce. Is often used to line plates, or in salads, soups or sandwiches. Wash well, drain. Will keep up to 2 weeks.

**Iceberg** — The familiar pale green, round-headed lettuce with crisp leaves and mild flavor.

**Romaine** — Loaf-shaped heads, with long, dark green, crisp leaves. Has a mild flavor, and is a familiar ingredient in Caesar salads. Has 3 times as much calcium, iron, and vitamin C, and 6 times as much vitamin A as iceberg lettuce.

## MACHÉ (Lamb's Lettuce)

Maché is a small flat plant, with pale to dark green leaves. It is a member of the valerian family, and has a bland flavor. Maché balances the flavor when mixed with bitter or peppery greens such as chicory. Choose fresh-looking, unblemished leaves. Wash. Trim roots and discard any discolored or damaged leaves. Available year round.

## MUSTARD GREENS

Large, dark green leaves with white midribs, or bright green with yellow-tinged, curly-edged leaves. Has a sharp flavor, great in tossed salads with other greens. The seeds of a certain variety are ground and used as mustard or whole in pickling. Will keep refrigerated about 2 weeks. Choose crisp green leaves with no limpness.

## PARSLEY

See herb list on page 65.

## PURSLANE

Has brittle red stalk and fleshy leaves, has a refreshing flavor and can be used in soups, salads, and sauces.

## SPINACH

Available year round, spinach is an excellent source of vitamins A and C, potassium, iron, and folic acid. Has thick, dark green leaves, crinkled or smooth. Give spinach a try, especially if you have based your dislike on canned spinach! Fresh spinach is tender and delicately flavored. When purchasing, check for unblemished leaves and short stems. Wash thoroughly in cold water, drain well, and store in plastic bag up to a week in refrigerator. DO NOT OVERCOOK. Spinach cooks in 5-8 minutes. Wonderful in a variety of dishes, and easy to prepare. Try it raw in salads, steamed with a dressing, or in quiche, pasta, sauces, stir-fry, even soups. Two pounds of fresh spinach will cook down to 2 cups and will serve 4 as a vegetable. In a salad, 1 pound will serve 4.

**Ceylon Spinach** — Bears a strong resemblance to flowering white cabbage, but has a milder taste. Choose large fleshy leaves, up to 7 inches long and 4 inches wide. Texture is similar to okra. Use raw in salads or add to stir-fry, soups, or stews.

**Chinese Spinach** — Commonly called Jacob's Coat or Amaranth. Peak season is April through November. Choose tender leaves with smooth stems. Wash and trim ends. Chinese spinach has a mild, sweet flavor that goes well with mixed greens in a salad or added to stir-fry or soup.

**New Zealand Spinach** (Summer Spinach) — The leaves are smaller than regular spinach, available May through October. Wash and trim stem ends, discard large stems. Great in salads.

**Winter Spinach** (Swamp Spinach) — Available April through October. Choose small, young leaves — the larger ones are tough. Wash and trim stem ends, discard any damaged leaves. Serve raw in salads or cooked.

# DRESSING YOUR GREENS

We often get into a rut when it comes to salad dressings and just reach for the same old bottled brand Mom used to serve. Don't fall into that rut! Oil and vinegar are two important ingredients to most salad lovers. Mustard, honey, herbs, or mayonnaise can be added for great variations on the basic oil and vinegar dressings. Try a variety of different vinegars and oils, too. To give you some idea of the varieties available, I have listed a few of the myriad varieties of oils and vinegars that are available to get your imagination going.

## OILS

**Safflower Oil** — Cholesterol-free, has a mild flavor and is light in color.

**Olive Oil** — Cholesterol-free. Olive oil is a monounsaturate. Color ranges from golden in color (with light flavor) to deep green (with a strong flavor). Virgin oil is obtained from the first pressing of the olives, and has the strongest taste.

**Avocado Oil** — This is a fairly new product, cholesterol-free (monounsaturated). Look for it in your market.

**Sesame Oil** — Whole sesame seeds are toasted and then mechanically pressed to release a rich, thick oil. A little goes a long way because of its strong flavor. Sesame oil is a highly regarded health food, easy to digest and versatile, great in stir-fry and salad dressings. Sesame oil is mostly unsaturated.

**Hot Chili Oil** — Spicy red chilies combined with vegetable oil for a strong "hot" flavor.

## VINEGARS

This low-carbohydrate, low-calorie condiment is an excellent choice for the health-conscious cook who is looking for ways to eliminate excess fat intake. There are many varieties:

**Red Wine Vinegar** — A favorite in salad dressings.

**White Wine Vinegar** — Light in color and flavor, great in salads.

**108**

**Cider Vinegar** — Has an apple cider base, producing a golden color and fruity flavor.

**Herb Vinegar** — Flavored with tarragon, rosemary, basil, sage, fennel, garlic, or other herbs. These vinegars make a delicious change in your salad dressings.

**Fruit Flavored Vinegar** — Made with raspberries, blueberries, cherries, strawberries, or your favorite fruit. These vinegars offer a distinctive, fruity flavor that is especially effective with fresh fruit salads.

**Rice Wine Vinegar** — This vinegar is made from rice wine and has a light flavor. Often used in Chinese dishes.

**Sherry Vinegar** — Made from sherry, used in both cooking and salads.

Use your imagination and make your own vinegar combinations. These combinations make great gifts for your family and friends.

---

### DITHIOTHIONES

Dithiothiones is not exactly a household word, not yet anyway. Dithiothiones, a group of substances found in broccoli, cabbage, cauliflower, Brussels sprouts and other so-called cruciferous vegetables, are hot items in cancer prevention research. Studies have shown that individuals whose diets include cabbage and other cruciferous vegetables have lower risk of cancer than individuals whose diets do not include cruciferous vegetables.

In a highly unusual research opportunity, three researchers are working together on a project sponsored by the American Institute for Cancer Research. Dr. Thomas W. Kensler at Johns Hopkins School of Hygiene and Public Health, Dr. John Groopman at Boston University School of Public Health, and Dr. Bill Roebuck at Dartmouth Medical School are studying exactly how dithiothiones protect against cancer. No specific recommendations can be made at this time, but ultimately this work may result in practical recommendations for people who are at high risk of getting cancer to include in their diets more food high in dithiothiones such as cabbage, Brussels sprouts, cauliflower, or broccoli.

*Source: The American Institute for Cancer Research Newsletter, Spring 1987, Issue 15.*

## OXALIC ACID CONTENT OF SELECTED VEGETABLES

**OXALIC ACID** — a chemical that can combine with calcium and prevent it from being absorbed.

| Vegetable | Oxalic acid (g/100g) | Vegetable | Oxalic acid (g/100g) |
|---|---|---|---|
| Amaranth | 1.09 | Kale | .02 |
| Asparagus | .13 | Lettuce | .33 |
| Beans, snap | .36 | Okra | .05 |
| Beet leaves | .61 | Onion | .05 |
| Broccoli | .19 | Parsley | 1.70 |
| Brussels sprouts | .36 | Parsnip | .04 |
| Cabbage | .10 | Peas | .05 |
| Carrot | .50 | Pepper | .04 |
| Cassava | 1.26 | Potato | .05 |
| Cauliflower | .15 | Purslane | 1.31 |
| Celery | .19 | Radish | .48 |
| Chicory | .21 | Rutabaga | .03 |
| Chives | 1.48 | Spinach | .97 |
| Collards | .45 | Squash | .02 |
| Coriander | .01 | Sweet potato | .24 |
| Corn, sweet | .01 | Tomato | .05 |
| Cucumbers | .02 | Turnip | .21 |
| Eggplant | .19 | Turnip greens | .05 |
| Endive | .11 | Watercress | .31 |
| Garlic | .36 | | |

*Source: Consumption of Foods: Vegetables and Vegetable Products, United States Department of Agriculture, Agriculture Handbook Number 8-11, Revised August 1984.*

## BRUSSELS SPROUTS

4 servings

1½ cups Brussels sprouts — halved
⅓ cup nitrate-free bacon — diced
3 garlic cloves — chopped
⅓ cup onion — chopped
½ cup green bell pepper — chopped
1 tomato — chopped
2-4 Tablespoons parmesan cheese
Pepper — optional

Steam Brussels sprouts until tender, but firm. In a skillet, combine bacon, garlic, and onion. Sauté for a couple of minutes, then add bell pepper. Sauté 2-3 minutes longer. Add steamed Brussels sprouts and cover. Let cook 3-4 minutes over medium-low heat (stir a couple of times). Add tomatoes, and stir again, sprinkle with cheese, and cover for a minute or so to melt the cheese slightly. Sprinkle with pepper.

## BOILED ASPARAGUS

4 servings

20-25 asparagus spears
2 Tablespoons fresh lemon juice
2 garlic cloves — pressed and minced
Lemon wedges for garnish

Trim off lower ends of all the spears; tie spears into a bundle with string. Bring 2 inches of water to a boil in a deep pot. Stand bundled spears upright in pot with spears up. Cover and let boil 4-6 minutes or until spears are tender; check by piercing with a fork. In a small dish, combine lemon juice and minced garlic. Drain asparagus and sprinkle with lemon juice/garlic mixture. Serve with lemon wedges.

## MUSHROOM PARSLEY POTATOES

2-4 servings

*2 Tablespoons olive oil*
*2 Tablespoons leeks — chopped*
*2 cups small red potatoes (with skin) — sliced*
*1 Tablespoon fresh parsley — chopped*
*1 cup fresh mushrooms — sliced*

In a skillet, heat oil. Add leeks and potatoes, and cook about 5 minutes over medium heat. Add parsley and mushrooms; continue cooking until potatoes are tender. Mix frequently to prevent sticking.

## BOB'S BAKED POTATO

1 serving

*1 baking potato*
*1 strip nitrate-free raw bacon*
*1 Tablespoon onion — diced*
*¼ teaspoon margarine*
*2 Tablespoons cheese — grated (optional)*

Cut potato halfway through and open up just enough to place bacon, onion, and margarine into center. Wrap tightly in foil and place on the grill or in the oven. Bake till tender. Discard bacon slices before serving. Top with grated cheese if desired.

# STUFFED MUSHROOMS FOR TWO

*4 large mushrooms*
*3 Tablespoons leeks — chopped*
*1 teaspoon unsalted butter*
*3 teaspoons parmesan cheese — grated*

Wash mushrooms and pat dry. Remove stems and centers of mushrooms, chop, and place in a skillet. Add leeks and butter, and sauté a few minutes. Spoon sautéed mushrooms into the 4 large caps, sprinkle with parmesan cheese. Broil until cheese melts, and serve.

# POTATO SHRIMP SALAD  4 servings

*6 small unpeeled red potatoes — boiled, chilled, and sliced*
*2 eggs — hard-boiled, chilled, and chopped*
*1 cup frozen baby early peas — rinsed briefly under warm water*
*1 cup (³/₄ pound) shrimp — rinsed, drained*
*2 Tablespoons green onion — chopped*
*2 Tablespoons fresh lemon juice*
*1 Tablespoon mayonnaise*
*¹/₄ cup 2% or nonfat milk*
*2 Tablespoons plain nonfat yogurt*

In a salad bowl, combine potatoes, eggs, peas, shrimp, and green onions. In a small bowl, combine lemon juice, mayonnaise, milk, and yogurt. Mix well and pour over potato mixture. Toss. Chill before serving.

## TABOULY SALAD

8 servings

1 - 7 ounce package of tabouly
3/4 cup water
1 cup tomato — chopped
1 Tablespoon olive oil
3 Tablespoons red wine vinegar
1 - 15 ounce can garbanzo beans
1 cup salmon — cooked and flaked

Mix all ingredients together and chill at least 1/2 hour before serving.

## POTATO SALAD

4 servings

6 small red potatoes — boiled, cooled, and chopped
3-4 eggs — hard-boiled, cooled, and chopped
4-6 red radishes — sliced thin
2 green onions — chopped
3 small sweet pickles — chopped
4-5 green olives — sliced
2 Tablespoons mayonnaise (Saffola polyunsaturated with
    no preservatives)
2 Tablespoons plain nonfat yogurt
Dab 2% milk
1 Tablespoon coarse brown mustard
Pepper
1 Tablespoon sweet pickle juice

In a bowl, combine potatoes, eggs, radishes, green onions, sweet pickles, and olives. Set aside. In a bowl, mix mayonnaise, yogurt, milk, mustard, pepper, and pickle juice. Pour over potato mixture. Toss and chill.

## POTATO SALAD WITH DILL AND TARRAGON

6 servings

*8-10 potatoes — cooked, chilled, and chopped*
*4 eggs — hard-boiled, cooled, and chopped*
*1/4 cup onion — chopped*
*10 green olives — chopped*
*1/2 cup plain nonfat yogurt*
*1/4 cup 2% or nonfat milk*
*1/4 cup mayonnaise*
*1 Tablespoon coarse mustard*
*7 black olives — sliced*
*Pepper*
*1/2 teaspoon dried dill*
*1/2 teaspoon dried tarragon*

Mix all ingredients well and chill.

# SPINACH-CORN SALAD

2-3 servings

*2-3 cups fresh spinach — chopped*
*2 green onions — chopped*
*1 cup whole kernel corn (canned or cut from fresh-cooked cob)*
*Pepper to taste*
*2 Tablespoons ranch-style dressing*

Toss spinach, green onion, corn, and pepper together. Chill and serve with ranch-style dressing.

# SPINACH TOSS SALAD

3-4 servings

*2 cups raw spinach leaves — washed and drained*
*¼ cup leeks — chopped*
*2 Tablespoons romano cheese — finely grated*
*2 Tablespoons unsalted sunflower seeds*
*10-12 black olives — sliced*
*1 Tablespoon olive oil*
*2 Tablespoons red wine vinegar*
*Pepper*
*1 Tablespoon fresh lemon juice*

Tear spinach into bite-sized pieces. Toss all ingredients and serve chilled.

**116**

## TOSSED GREEN SALAD

*1 cup romaine lettuce — chopped*
*1 cup fresh spinach — chopped*
*1 cup fresh mushrooms — sliced*
*¼ cup leeks — chopped*
*¼ cup red bell pepper — sliced thin*
*1 tomato — cut in half and sliced*
*3 Tablespoons parmesan cheese — grated*

In salad bowl, toss together romaine and spinach leaves. Top with mushrooms, leeks, bell pepper, and tomato slices. Sprinkle cheese over top. Toss at table with favorite dressing before serving.

Note: Cauliflower and green onions make great additions to this salad.

## BEETS AND BEANS SALAD

Approximately 2½ cups

*1 cup canned lima or garbanzo beans*
*1 cup cooked beets — chilled and sliced (or use canned beets)*
*2 Tablespoons leeks — chopped*
*¼ cup onion — sliced*
*1 Tablespoon olive oil*
*2 Tablespoons tarragon vinegar*
*1 teaspoon fresh parsley — chopped (optional)*

Mix well. Toss and serve.

# SPINACH CHICKEN SALAD

*2 cups fresh spinach — rinsed and drained*
*1 cup fresh mushrooms — cleaned and sliced*
*1 fresh tomato — chopped or cut into wedges*
*½ cup green bell pepper — sliced thin*
*1 Tablespoon olive oil*
*1½ Tablespoons tarragon vinegar*
*2 Tablespoons fresh lemon juice*
*Pepper (optional)*
*3 Tablespoons parmesan cheese — grated*
*⅓ cup whole wheat flour*
*2 teaspoons fresh rosemary — diced*
*2 chicken breasts — remove skin, de-bone*
*1 teaspoon olive oil*
*½ teaspoon sesame seed oil*
*2 Tablespoons fresh lemon juice*
*2 Tablespoons sesame seeds*
*3 Tablespoons tarragon vinegar*

In a salad bowl, toss spinach (torn into bite-sized pieces), mushrooms, tomato, and green bell pepper. In a small bowl, combine 1 Tablespoon olive oil, 1½ Tablespoons tarragon vinegar, and 2 Tablespoons fresh lemon juice. Mix well. Pepper is optional. Pour mixture over tossed spinach and mix well. Sprinkle with grated cheese, and chill.

In a bowl, combine flour and rosemary. Cut chicken into strips, dredge in flour mixture. In a skillet, heat 1 teaspoon olive oil, ½ teaspoon sesame seed oil, and 2 Tablespoons lemon juice over medium heat. Add chicken strips, sprinkling with sesame seeds. Cook, browning strips on both sides, for 4-5 minutes. Add 3 Tablespoons tarragon vinegar, and continue cooking 4-5 minutes longer, until chicken is done.

Remove from heat. Arrange chicken strips on top of chilled salad and serve.

# SPINACH-CAULIFLOWER SALAD

2-3 servings

*2 cups fresh spinach leaves*
*³/₄ cup cauliflower florets*
*1 small tomato — sliced*
*½ teaspoon sesame seed oil*
*2 Tablespoons tarragon vinegar*
*1 Tablespoon light mayonnaise*
*½ teaspoon dried basil*

Rinse and drain spinach and cauliflower. In a salad bowl, combine spinach, cauliflower, and tomato slices. In a small bowl, mix sesame seed oil, tarragon, vinegar, mayonnaise, and basil. Pour over spinach, toss and serve.

## SPINACH-BELGIAN ENDIVE
## SALAD

4 servings

$^1/_2$ cup Belgian endive — rinsed and drained
1 cup fresh spinach — rinsed, drained, and ripped into bite-sized
    pieces
1 cup leaf lettuce — rinsed, drained, and ripped into bite-sized
    pieces
$^3/_4$ cup fresh mushrooms — sliced
$^1/_2$ cup leeks — chopped
$^1/_3$ cup red bell pepper — cut into thin strips
$^1/_3$ cup yellow bell pepper — cut into thin strips

In a salad bowl, combine all ingredients and chill before serving.
Serve with your favorite salad dressing.


## SPINACH SALAD
## WITH CILANTRO

3-4 servings

2 cups fresh spinach — chopped
$^1/_3$ cup onion — sliced thin
1 tomato — chopped
2-3 Tablespoons fresh cilantro — chopped
1 cup fresh mushrooms — sliced
2 Tablespoons plain nonfat yogurt
$1^1/_2$ teaspoons mayonnaise
2 Tablespoons red wine vinegar
Pepper

In a bowl, combine spinach, onion, tomato, cilantro, and fresh mushrooms. In a small bowl, combine yogurt, mayonnaise, vinegar, and pepper, and mix well. Pour yogurt mixture over spinach mixture, toss, chill, and serve.

---

# CHEESE FONDUE FOR TWO

*1 large garlic clove*
*$1/3$ - $1/2$ pound lowfat swiss cheese*
*2 Tablespoons unbleached white flour*
*1 cup white wine*
*1 teaspoon lemon juice (optional)*
*$1/4$ teaspoon nutmeg — freshly grated*
*Dippers — French bread, pickles, or vegetables*

Cut garlic clove in half, rub the inside of fondue pot, and discard clove. Grate cheese. Add white flour to cheese and mix well. Add wine to fondue pot and heat until it bubbles. Add lemon juice and cheese by the handful (stirring until smooth after each addition). Add nutmeg last, and mix until fondue is smooth and creamy (add more cheese if necessary).
Serve hot with cubed French bread, pickles, or a variety of vegetables such as jicama, turnips, zucchini, olives, cherry tomatoes, mushrooms, broccoli (to name a few).

# SALAMI-ASPARAGUS SALAD                2 servings

*¼ cup cooked asparagus — chopped*
*½ cup apple — chopped*
*¼ cup salami — chopped*
*1 small carrot — grated*
*1 Tablespoon olive oil*
*1 Tablespoon tarragon vinegar*
*3 Tablespoons plain nonfat yogurt*
*2 Tablespoons parmesan cheese — freshly grated*
*Pepper*

In a bowl, mix asparagus, apple, salami, and carrot. Set aside. In a second bowl, mix olive oil, vinegar, and yogurt, pour over asparagus mixture, and toss. Sprinkle with cheese and pepper. Toss again before serving.

# 4 BEAN SALAD          Approximately 3⅓ cups salad

*½ cup garbanzo beans — cooked or canned*
*½ cup red kidney beans — cooked or canned*
*½ cup large (butter) lima beans — cooked or canned*
*½ cup small green lima beans — cooked or canned*
*½ cup onion — sliced thin*
*¼ cup fresh chives — chopped*
*½ cup fresh mushrooms — sliced*
*3 Tablespoons olive oil or favorite unsaturated oil*
*3 Tablespoons red wine vinegar*

Toss all ingredients and chill. This salad tastes great left overnight to marinate. (See page 290 for bean cooking chart.)

# FAST & EASY GARBANZO BEAN-CARROT SALAD

4 servings

1 - 15 ounce can garbanzo beans — rinsed
1 cup carrots — shredded
1 Tablespoon olive oil
1½ Tablespoons red wine vinegar
½ teaspoon fennel seed — optional
2 Tablespoons mayonnaise (I use Hollywood mayonnaise with safflower oil. It is low in cholesterol and salt and has no preservatives.)

Combine all ingredients, toss well, and chill before serving.

# CARROT SALAD

4 servings

3 carrots — grated
¼ cup leek — chopped
1 cup pineapple — chopped and drained (fresh or canned)
½ green apple — grated
¼ cup raisins
¼ cup sunflower seeds (unsalted)
3 Tablespoons plain nonfat yogurt
1 Tablespoon safflower mayonnaise — no preservatives

Mix all ingredients. Serve chilled.

# CARROT-APRICOT SALAD

4 servings

*1 cup carrots — grated*
*1 teaspoon fresh lemon juice*
*³/₄-1 cup fresh apricots — chopped*
*2 Tablespoons unsalted sunflower seeds*
*1 Tablespoon honey*
*¼ cup plain nonfat yogurt*
*½ teaspoon poppy seeds — optional*

In a bowl, mix together carrots, lemon juice, apricots and sunflower seeds.
In a small bowl, mix honey and yogurt. Add to carrot mixture and toss until well mixed. Chill. Sprinkle with poppy seeds (optional).

# CABBAGE-GARBANZO BEANS-CARROT SALAD

4 servings

*²/₃ cup carrot — grated*
*1 cup cabbage — sliced thin*
*1 - 15 ounce can garbanzo beans — drained (or 1 cup cooked beans)*
*½ cup leeks — chopped*
*1 Tablespoon light mayonnaise*
*2 Tablespoons plain nonfat yogurt*
*2 Tablespoons red wine vinegar*
*Pepper*
*¼ teaspoon dried mint — optional*

**124**

Combine carrots, cabbage, beans and leeks in a salad bowl. In a small bowl, mix mayonnaise, yogurt, red wine vinegar, and pepper. Pour mixture over carrot/cabbage mixture and toss well, sprinkle with mint, chill, and toss again before serving.

---

## VEGETABLE-TUNA SALAD                4 servings

This salad is a healthy lunch.

*³/₄ cup yellow bell pepper — cut into thin strips*
*³/₄ cup red bell pepper — cut into thin strips*
*³/₄ cup green bell pepper — cut into thin strips*
*¹/₂ cup celery — sliced*
*³/₄ cups cauliflower — broken into florets*
*³/₄ cup leeks — chopped*
*1 - 6 ounce can tuna — drained (water packed)*
*2 teaspoons red wine vinegar*
*1 Tablespoon plain nonfat yogurt*
*1 Tablespoon mayonnaise*
*1 Tablespoon fresh lemon juice*
*2 teaspoons fresh dill — chopped*
*Pepper — optional*

In a large bowl, combine bell peppers, celery, cauliflower, leeks, and drained tuna. Toss. In a small bowl, combine vinegar, yogurt, mayonnaise, lemon juice, dill, and pepper. Mix well. Pour dressing over vegetables and toss until mixed well. Chill and serve.

## GARBANZO-TUNA SALAD
## IN A PITA

4 pitas

*1 - 15 ounce can garbanzo beans — or 1 cup cooked*
*½ cup tomato — halved and then sliced*
*2 Tablespoons green onion — chopped*
*¾ cup fresh mushrooms — washed and sliced*
*1 - 6½ ounce can tuna (water packed) — drained*
*1 Tablespoon red wine vinegar*
*1 large garlic clove — pressed*
*1 Tablespoon fresh lemon juice*
*1½ Tablespoons mayonnaise*
*2 Tablespoons plain nonfat yogurt*
*4 pita breads*
*Garnish — 4 slices of cheese*
*4 leaves of spinach or lettuce*

Mix all ingredients and chill. Open pitas, fill with mixture, and serve. Add a slice of cheese and leaf of spinach as garnish.

Note: Salmon can be substituted for the tuna. Sprouts are also great in this sandwich.

# GARBANZO BEANS & RED CABBAGE SALAD

4 servings

*1½ cups red cabbage — sliced thin*
*1 - 15 ounce can garbanzo beans*
*⅓ cup leeks — chopped*
*2 Tablespoons fresh orange juice*
*2 Tablespoons fresh lemon juice*
*2½ Tablespoons plain lowfat yogurt*
*1½ Tablespoons mayonnaise*
*Pepper — to taste*

In a bowl, toss together the red cabbage, beans, leek, orange juice, and lemon juice. In a small bowl, combine the yogurt and mayonnaise. Mix well. Pour over cabbage. Sprinkle with pepper and toss. Chill and serve.

# GARBANZO BEANS WITH BASIL

4 servings

*2 - 15 ounce cans garbanzo beans (or fresh soaked)*
*1 cup tomato — sliced*
*1½ Tablespoons fresh basil — chopped fine*
*3 Tablespoons green onion — chopped*
*1 Tablespoon olive oil*
*1½ Tablespoons red wine vinegar*
*2 Tablespoons fresh lime juice*

Toss all ingredients in a salad bowl, and chill at least ½ hour before serving.

# BAKED GARLIC TOMATOES

4 servings

4 tomatoes
2 garlic cloves — pressed and minced
1 Tablespoon parmesan cheese — grated
1 Tablespoon romano cheese — grated
1 Tablespoon jarlsberg cheese — grated
Pepper (optional)

Preheat oven to 375°

Cut tomatoes in half. Place in a baking dish with cut side up. Rub the top of each tomato half with garlic. Combine the cheeses and place on top, then sprinkle with pepper. Bake for 5-8 minutes, or until cheese melts and tomatoes are hot.

# BAKED TOMATOES

4 servings

4 medium-sized tomatoes
Pepper (optional)
1 teaspoon fresh lemon juice
2 teaspoons dijon mustard
2 Tablespoons dry bread crumbs — finely ground
½ teaspoon onion — minced
3 Tablespoons parmesan cheese — grated

Preheat oven to 375°

Cut tomatoes in half. Place in a baking dish with cut side up. Sprinkle each with pepper. In a small bowl, combine lemon juice, dijon mustard, bread crumbs, and onions. Top each tomato half with breadcrumb mixture. Sprinkle with cheese. Bake 8-10 minutes, or until tomatoes are hot.

# GARDEN SALAD

4 servings

*³/₄ cup red cabbage — sliced thin*
*¹/₂ cup red bell pepper — cut into thin strips*
*³/₄ cup yellow squash — sliced*
*1 cup fresh mushrooms — sliced*
*¹/₄ cup fennel bulb — sliced thin*
*¹/₄ cup jicama — cut into thin strips*
*4 romaine lettuce leaves*

In a salad bowl, combine all ingredients except romaine lettuce, and toss. Line 4 salad plates with romaine lettuce, place tossed vegetables on each. Serve with your favorite dressing or use Fennel Dressing on page 136.

# BROCCOLI-SPROUT SALAD

4 servings

*2 garlic cloves — mince and rub on inside of salad bowl*
*3 cups broccoli — steamed and chilled*
*³/₄ cup onion — sliced thin*
*1 cup alfalfa sprouts (or your favorite sprout) — rinsed and drained*
*2 Tablespoons fresh lemon juice*

Toss all ingredients. Chill. Serve plain or with a favorite dressing. Optional: ¹/₄ cup unsalted sunflower seeds.

## BOK CHOY AND BROCCOLI STIR-FRY

4 servings

*2 teaspoons olive oil*
*⅓ cup onion — chopped*
*¼ cup leeks — chopped*
*1½ cups broccoli — chopped*
*1 Tablespoon soy sauce*
*2 Tablespoons fresh lemon juice*
*2 cups bok choy — sliced*

In a skillet, heat oil. Add onions, and leeks. Sauté for a minute or so. Add broccoli, soy sauce, and lemon juice and sauté for 5 minutes. Add bok choy and cook 3-4 minutes longer.

## BROCCOLI WITH SESAME SEEDS

4 servings

*1 bunch broccoli (about 1½ pounds)*
*1 Tablespoon olive oil*
*2 Tablespoons oyster sauce*
*1 Tablespoon low-sodium soy sauce*
*¼ cup water*
*1½ Tablespoons sesame seeds*

Trim outer leaves and tough ends of stalks of broccoli. Cut stalk and florets into 2-inch lengths, then into thin slices. Heat oil in a skillet or wok till hot. Stir in broccoli and stir-fry about 5 minutes (or until broccoli turns bright green). Add oyster sauce, soy sauce, and water. Bring to a boil and let simmer about 5 more minutes.

Meanwhile, toast sesame seeds in a small skillet over low heat, stirring constantly until browned. Remove from heat and stir into broccoli mixture. Serve warm.

Note: Oyster sauce can be found in Asian section at market.

---

# JICAMA TOSSED SALAD                    4 servings

Nice and crunchy.

*¹/₂ cup jicama — peeled and cut into thin strips*
*¹/₂ cup carrots — grated*
*¹/₂ cup fresh mushrooms — sliced*
*2 Tablespoons onion — diced*
*¹/₂ cup red bell pepper — cut into thin strips*

**DRESSING**
*1 teaspoon sesame seed oil*
*1 Tablespoon olive oil*
*2 Tablespoons tarragon white wine vinegar*
*2 Tablespoons fresh lemon juice*

In a bowl, combine jicama, carrots, mushrooms, onion, and red bell pepper.
In a small bowl, combine sesame oil, olive oil, vinegar, and lemon juice. Pour over vegetables and toss well. Chill.

# BROCCOLI AND CAULIFLOWER SALAD

4 servings

*1 cup broccoli florets — steamed*
*1 cup raw cauliflower florets*
*3 Tablespoons unsalted sunflower seeds — optional*
*¼ cup raisins*
*1 Tablespoon mayonnaise*
*3 Tablespoons plain nonfat yogurt*
*1½ teaspoons honey*
*2 Tablespoons fresh lemon juice*
*2 garlic cloves — chopped and pressed*

In a salad bowl, combine broccoli, cauliflower, sunflower seeds, and raisins. In a small bowl, mix mayonnaise, yogurt, honey, lemon juice, and garlic. Mix well and pour over broccoli mixture. Toss and chill.

# SWEET POTATOES

4 servings

*3 medium sweet potatoes — parboiled and peeled*
*1½ Tablespoons olive oil*
*½ cup bran*
*2 Tablespoons brown sugar*

Boil sweet potatoes until tender, not mushy. Drain. Slice about ½ inch thick. Coat each slice with bran. In a skillet, heat olive oil. Place sweet potatoes in skillet and brown on both sides. Sprinkle tops with brown sugar on the top and serve warm.

# TOSSED GREEN SALAD
# WITH BREAD STICKS
2-3 servings

*1 cup romaine lettuce*
*1 cup bibb lettuce*
*¼ cup unsalted sunflower seeds*
*½ cup red onion — sliced*
*Fresh sprouts*
*Thin bread sticks*

Wash and drain romaine and bibb lettuce. Break into bite-sized pieces. In a glass bowl, combine lettuce, sunflower seeds, and onion slices. Place sprouts over top. Tuck bread sticks into salad. Just before serving, break sticks into salad and serve with favorite Italian salad dressing.

## CHRISTINE'S GREEN BEAN, ALMOND AND MUSHROOM SALAD

4-6 servings

*1 pound green beans, trimmed and cut into 2-inch lengths*
*1 cup basic Italian salad dressing*
*2 cups fresh mushrooms — sliced*
*½ cup slivered almonds*
*½ cup green onions — chopped fine*
*1-2 Tablespoons fresh parsley — minced (optional)*

Steam the beans until bright green and crisp-tender. Rinse under cold water to stop the cooking. Toss beans with salad dressing and refrigerate for 1-2 hours.

Just before serving, add mushrooms, almonds, green onions, and parsley with green beans mixture. Toss well and serve.

## VEGETABLE AND PASTA SALAD WITH ANCHOVY DRESSING

4-6 servings

*2 cups spiral pasta (spinach or whole wheat) — cooked, drained, and chilled*
*⅓ cup red bell pepper — cut into thin strips*
*1 cup broccoli florets — steamed and chilled*
*¾ cup fresh mushrooms — sliced*
*¼ cup leeks — chopped*
*1 - 2 ounce can of anchovies — drained (save anchovy oil)*
*1 teaspoon anchovy oil (drained from can)*
*2 garlic cloves — minced*
*1 Tablespoon fresh lemon juice*

**134**

*3 Tablespoons plain nonfat yogurt*
*1 teaspoon dijon mustard*
*1 Tablespoon mayonnaise*

In a salad bowl, combine cooked pasta, red bell pepper, broccoli, mushrooms, and leeks. Toss and set aside.

In a blender, combine drained anchovies, 1 teaspoon anchovy oil, garlic, lemon juice, yogurt, mustard, and mayonnaise. Blend until smooth. Pour anchovy sauce over pasta and vegetables, toss, chill, and serve.

---

# CUCUMBER YOGURT SAUCE

Approximately 1 cup

*¹/₂ cup cucumber — peeled and shredded*
*¹/₂ cup plain nonfat yogurt*
*1 Tablespoon green onion — chopped fine*
*¹/₂ teaspoon fresh parsley — chopped fine*
*¹/₂ teaspoon fresh dill — chopped fine*
*2 garlic cloves — pressed and chopped*
*1 teaspoon red wine vinegar*
*¹/₂ teaspoon fresh lemon juice*

Shred cucumber and drain on a paper towel. In a bowl, combine cucumber and remaining ingredients, mixing well. Chill at least 1 hour. Very tasty with vegetables or seafood.

# FENNEL DRESSING

Approximately ½ cup

3 Tablespoons olive oil
¼ cup water
3 Tablespoons red wine vinegar
1 teaspoon fresh lemon juice
½ teaspoon dijon mustard
2 garlic cloves — sliced
¼ teaspoon fennel seeds — crushed

Combine all ingredients and whip. Cover and chill at least 2 hours.

# FRENCH DRESSING

Approximately 2 cups

¼ cup oil
¼ cup vinegar
½ teaspoon paprika
⅓ cup honey
¼ cup ketchup
2 Tablespoons fresh lemon juice
2 Tablespoons grated onion
¼ teaspoon salt — optional

Blend well and chill.

# LUCY'S WHITE SAUCE

**THIN SAUCE**
*2 teaspoons margarine or unsalted butter*
*1 Tablespoon flour*
*Pinch of salt*
*1 cup 2% or nonfat milk*

**MEDIUM SAUCE**
*1½ Tablespoons margarine or unsalted butter*
*2 Tablespoons flour*
*Pinch of salt*
*1 cup 2% or nonfat milk*

**THICK SAUCE**
*2 Tablespoons margarine or unsalted butter*
*3 Tablespoons flour*
*Pinch of salt*
*1 cup 2% or nonfat milk*

In a saucepan, melt margarine or butter. Add flour and salt and blend until smooth. Add milk, all at once, and stir constantly until sauce becomes thick and smooth.

This sauce is great for creamed cauliflower, carrots, peas, beans, even potatoes.

# AL'S HORSERADISH SAUCE

*3½ Tablespoons grated horseradish root*
*1 Tablespoon white vinegar*
*¼ teaspoon pepper*
*4 Tablespoons whipping cream — whipped*

Mix horseradish root, vinegar, and pepper. Fold into whipped cream. Chill.

# DRIED TOMATO-MUSHROOM QUICHE

4-6 servings

*¼ cup dried tomatoes — diced*
*1 partially baked pie crust (see page 270)*
*1 Tablespoon olive oil*
*½ cup fresh mushrooms — chopped*
*½ cup leeks — diced*
*4 eggs — discard 2 yolks*
*3 Tablespoons parmesan cheese — grated*
*1 teaspoon dijon mustard*
*1½ cups 2% milk*
*Garnish — 3 strips leek, 3 strips dried tomato*

Preheat oven to 350°
Spread dried tomatoes over the bottom of a partially baked pie crust. In a skillet, heat olive oil. Add mushrooms and leeks, and sauté for a few minutes. Remove from heat and spread mixture over bottom of crust. In blender, place eggs (using only 2 yolks), cheese, mustard, and milk. Blend well and pour mixture into pie crust. Lay 3 strips leek and 3 strips of dried tomato on top for design. Bake for 35-40 minutes.

**138**

# EGGS AND MUSHROOMS

*1 Tablespoon olive oil*
*½ cup onion — chopped*
*1 garlic clove — minced*
*2 jalapeño chili peppers — chopped*
*½ cup green bell pepper — sliced*
*8-10 mushrooms — sliced thick*
*5 eggs — discard 3 yolks*
*½ cup nonfat milk*
*Pepper to taste*
*Pinch of dried cumin — ground*
*Pinch of dried oregano*
*½ cup monterey jack cheese — grated*
*1 tomato — chopped large*

In a skillet, combine olive oil, onion, garlic, and chili peppers, and sauté about 3-5 minutes. Add green bell pepper and cook a few minutes longer. Add mushrooms and cook a few more minutes. In a bowl, mix eggs, milk, and spices, and add to skillet. Cook, stirring constantly, about 3-4 minutes. Add grated cheese and tomato. Cook until done to personal taste (wet or dry).

# EGGS WITH ZUCCHINI

2 servings

*1 Tablespoon olive oil*
*¼ cup onion — chopped*
*1 garlic clove — crushed*
*1 cup zucchini — sliced*
*3 eggs — discard 2 yolks*
*½ cup nonfat milk*
*Pinch of ground cumin*
*½ cup jarlsberg cheese — grated*
*Pepper to taste*

In a skillet, heat oil and sauté onion and garlic. Add zucchini and cook a few minutes until onions are tender. In a small bowl, beat eggs. Add milk and cumin, mix together, and add to skillet. Add cheese and pepper. Scramble to your taste, stirring frequently. Serve with toast.

# SANDY'S SPINACH-MUSHROOM SAUCE

Approximately 5 cups

1 Tablespoon olive oil
3 garlic cloves — chopped and pressed
¼ cup onion — chopped
1 fresh bunch of spinach — washed, drained, and chopped
4 cups fresh mushrooms — quartered
2 teaspoons dried marjoram
4 teaspoons dried basil or 3 Tablespoons fresh basil —chopped
1 teaspoon dried thyme
1 - 28 ounce can tomatoes
1 - 6 ounce can tomato paste
1 - 15 ounce can tomato sauce

In a saucepan, heat oil. Add garlic and onion. Sauté until onions are tender. Add spinach. Cover and cook 3-4 minutes. Add mushrooms, marjoram, basil, and thyme, and sauté about 3 minutes. Add tomatoes, tomato paste, and tomato sauce. Simmer 30-45 minutes or, if desired, just heat through and eat immediately.
This sauce is great over pasta or vegetables, or on a pizza crust.

Note: If you dislike basil, or are not familiar with it, cut back on the amount used.

# SAUCE III — FAST AND EASY

Approximately 5 cups

3 garlic cloves — diced
3 Tablespoons leeks — chopped
1 Tablespoon olive oil
½ cup onion — chopped
1 cup mushrooms — washed and quartered
1 bunch fresh spinach — washed, drained, and chopped
2 - 6½ ounce cans clams with juice
1 cup favorite commercial spaghetti sauce
1 cup tomato — chopped
Pepper
1 cup raw broccoli — chopped
1 teaspoon dried basil
1 teaspoon dried thyme
1 teaspoon dried oregano

In a saucepan, combine garlic, leeks, olive oil, and onion; sauté 2-3 minutes. Add quartered mushrooms and chopped spinach; simmer 2-3 minutes. Add clams and clam juice, spaghetti sauce, tomatoes, pepper, broccoli, basil, thyme, and oregano. Simmer 30-45 minutes. Serve over vegetables or favorite pasta.

# RAOUL'S MARINATED SALAD

4 servings

1½ cups spinach egg noodles
8 green olives — sliced
5 marinated artichoke hearts — chopped into chunks
1 Tablespoon pimientos — chopped
1 cup salmon — fresh cooked or canned
¾ cup carrots — cooked and cut into thin strips
1 teaspoon dried oregano
¼ cup onion — minced
1 Tablespoon fresh parsley — chopped
2 Tablespoons olive oil
1 Tablespoon lemon juice — fresh-squeezed
¼ teaspoon Worcestershire sauce
1 large garlic clove pressed — discard pulp
2 Tablespoons white tarragon vinegar

Cook spinach egg noodles till tender. Drain and cool. Mix all other ingredients well. Refrigerate at least 2 hours or overnight.

# EGGPLANT-TOFU CASSEROLE  6-8 servings

1 eggplant, medium
4 Tablespoons olive oil
1 cup onion — chopped
3 Tablespoons tomato paste
1/4 cup sherry or white wine
1/2 cup water
2 green onions — chopped
1 cup fresh mushrooms — sliced
1/8 teaspoon cinnamon
1/4 teaspoon nutmeg
1 cup lowfat cottage cheese, small curd
1 cup plain tofu — drain and cut into cubes
2 Tablespoons soybean margarine
3 Tablespoons flour
2 cups nonfat milk
2 eggs — beaten
1 cup bread crumbs, fine
1/2 cup parmesan cheese — grated

Preheat oven to 375°

Peel eggplant and slice into 1/2-inch thick strips. In a skillet, brown eggplant quickly in 2 Tablespoons oil and set aside. In a saucepan, sauté onions in remaining oil. Add tomato paste, sherry, water, green onions, mushrooms, cinnamon, and nutmeg. Simmer on very low heat. Stir frequently until most of the liquid is absorbed (about 10-15 minutes).

Combine cottage cheese and tofu cubes. Set aside.

In a small bowl, blend margarine and flour together until smooth. Set aside. Bring 2 cups of milk to a boil, slowly adding margarine and flour mixture, stirring constantly. When thick and smooth, remove from heat and cool slightly. Stir in cottage cheese mixture and beaten eggs. Mix well.

Sprinkle the bottom of an 11x14 baking dish with bread crumbs. Alternate layers of eggplant and tomato sauce. Sprinkle each layer with cheese and bread crumbs. Pour cottage cheese mixture over top. Bake for 1 hour or until golden brown. Cool before serving. Reheat and serve the next day. Makes great leftovers.

# VEGETARIAN LASAGNA

6-8 servings

1 Tablespoon olive oil
1 cup onion — sliced
2 garlic cloves — chopped
1/4 cup green onions — chopped
1/2 cup green pepper — chopped
1 cup zucchini — sliced
1 cup celery — sliced
1 cup carrots — grated
7 stalks raw asparagus — chopped
1 - 9 ounce can tomatoes
1 - 6 ounce can tomato paste
1 - 8 ounce can lima beans — drained
Pepper
1 Tablespoon dried thyme
1 Tablespoon dried basil
1 teaspoon ground cumin
Couple dashes cayenne pepper
3/4 pound lowfat mozzarella cheese — grated
1/2 cup parmesan cheese — grated
1 pound lowfat cottage cheese — small curd
1/4 cup fresh parsley — chopped
1 eggplant, small — peeled and sliced (raw)
1 cup fresh mushrooms — sliced
1/2 pound whole wheat lasagna noodles — uncooked

Preheat oven to 350°

In a skillet, heat olive oil and sauté onion and garlic. Add green onions, green peppers, zucchini, celery, carrots, asparagus, tomatoes, tomato paste, lima beans, pepper, thyme, basil, cumin, and cayenne. Simmer sauce, uncovered, approximately 35 minutes. Meanwhile, in a bowl, mix mozzarella, parmesan, and cottage cheeses, and parsley. Set aside. In another bowl, mix eggplant and mushrooms.

**146**

Layer whole wheat lasagna noodles (uncooked); eggplant and mushrooms; cheese mixture; sauce; repeat. Bake for 30-35 minutes. Cool 5-10 minutes before slicing.

## *ZUCCHINI SPAGHETTI SAUCE*

Approximately 6$^1/_2$ cups

*1 Tablespoon oil*
*1 cup onion — chopped*
*2 large garlic cloves — chopped*
*2 cups zucchini — sliced thick*
*1 cup fresh mushrooms — quartered*
*1 cup favorite commercial spaghetti sauce*
*1 - 15 ounce can stewed tomatoes*
*1 cup water*
*Pepper*
*$^1/_2$ teaspoon dried basil*
*1 teaspoon dried green oregano*
*$^1/_2$ teaspoon dried thyme*
*1 tomato — chopped*
*$^1/_4$ cup sherry*

Heat oil and sauté onion and garlic. Add the rest of the ingredients and simmer about 1 hour.

Note: Cut zucchini large so they don't disappear.

# CILANTRO LASAGNA

6 servings

2 teaspoons olive oil
2 large garlic cloves — chopped
3/4 cup onion — chopped
1 teaspoon dried thyme
1/4 cup fresh cilantro — rinse, drain, and trim stems — chopped
1 - 14 1/2 ounce can tomatoes
1/2 cup water
1 - 6 ounce can tomato paste
1 Tablespoon fresh lemon juice
1 1/2 cups zucchini — sliced (about 3 small zucchini)
3/4 cup fresh mushrooms — sliced
Pepper (optional)
1 pound firm plain tofu — drained
1 1/2 cups lowfat mozzarella cheese — grated
2 Tablespoons fresh cilantro — rinsed and chopped
1 Tablespoon fresh parsley — chopped
1 teaspoon dried thyme
1 teaspoon dried oregano
Pepper
1 pound whole wheat or spinach lasagna noodles — raw
1/4 cup parmesan cheese — grated

Preheat oven to 350°

In a saucepan, heat oil. Add garlic, onion, and 1 teaspoon thyme. Sauté a minute or so. Add 1/4 cup cilantro, tomatoes, water, tomato paste, lemon juice, zucchini, mushrooms, and pepper. Simmer over medium to medium-low heat until sauce thickens. Meanwhile, drain tofu. In a bowl combine tofu, mozzarella cheese, 2 Tablespoons cilantro, parsley, 1 teaspoon thyme, 1 teaspoon oregano, and pepper. Mix well. Place a couple of Tablespoons of sauce in the bottom of an 8x11 baking dish, then place a layer of lasagna noodles (slightly overlapping), then spread 1/2 of tofu-cheese mixture on top of noodles, followed by a layer of sauce, layer of

148

noodles, layer of tofu-cheese mixture, and remaining sauce. Bake for 30 minutes. Sprinkle with $^1/_4$ cup parmesan cheese and bake 5 more minutes. Remove from oven and let sit 3-5 minutes before cutting and serving.

---

# ANOTHER SPAGHETTI SAUCE
Approximately 4$^1/_2$ cups

*1 Tablespoon olive oil*
*$^3/_4$ cup onion — chopped*
*5 garlic cloves — chopped*
*$^1/_4$ cup leeks — chopped*
*2 Tablespoons dried basil*
*1 Tablespoon fresh chives — optional*
*1 pound ground beef*
*1 cup cooked garbanzo beans (or 1 - 15$^1/_2$ ounce can)*
*1 - 15 ounce can salt-free tomatoes*
*1 - 8 ounce can tomato sauce*
*$^1/_2$ cup water*
*$^1/_2$ cup sliced black olives*

In a large saucepan, heat oil. Add onions, garlic, leeks, basil, and chives. Sauté 2-3 minutes on medium-low heat. In a skillet, brown ground beef. Add to onion mixture. Add garbanzo beans, tomatoes, tomato sauce, water, and black olives. Mix well and simmer 20-45 minutes. Wonderful over pasta or vegetables.

# DUFFY'S BAKED EGGPLANT

4-6 servings

## TOMATO SAUCE

*1 cup onion*
*2 garlic cloves — chopped fine*
*1 Tablespoon olive oil (more if needed)*
*1 cup carrot — grated*
*³/4 cup green bell pepper — chopped*
*1 or 2 bay leaves*
*2 teaspoons dried oregano*
*1 teaspoon dried thyme*
*¹/2 teaspoon dried basil*
*2-4 Tablespoons fresh parsley — chopped*
*3 - 14¹/2 ounce cans whole tomatoes*
*1 - 6 ounce can tomato sauce*
*Pepper*
*2 Tablespoons fresh lemon juice*

Preheat oven to 350°

Sauté onion and garlic in olive oil until onions are tender. Add carrots, green bell pepper, bay leaf, oregano, thyme, basil, and parsley. Stir well. Add tomatoes, tomato sauce, pepper, and lemon juice. Let simmer ¹/2 hour. Remove bay leaf.

Meanwhile, prepare 3 bowls for dipping eggplant.

1. *1 cup whole wheat flour*
2. *2 eggs — beaten*
   *¹/4 cup 2% milk*
3. *2¹/2 cups cracker crumbs*
   *¹/2 teaspoon pepper*
   *¹/2 teaspoon oregano*

*1 large eggplant — peeled and cut into ¹/₄-inch rounds*
*³/₄ cup parmesan cheese — grated*
*¹/₂ cup lowfat mozzarella cheese — grated*

Dip slices of eggplant into flour, then egg mixture. Coat completely with cracker mixture. Layer in a 9x13 baking dish. Slices may overlap but not cover each other completely. Sprinkle each layer with tomato sauce and parmesan cheese (reserve some parmesan cheese for topping). Cover tightly with foil and bake 30-45 minutes, or until fork pierces middle slices easily. Remove from oven, top with mozzarella cheese and remaining parmesan cheese. Return to oven just until cheese melts.

Note: Because the sizes of eggplants vary so much, you may need 1¹/₂ eggplants for this dish to build sufficient layers.

## SNOWPEAS WITH PINENUTS STIR-FRY

3-4 servings

*1 Tablespoon oil*
*3 large garlic cloves — chopped*
*1 teaspoon fresh ginger — diced*
*¹/₄ cup pinenuts*
*2 cups snowpeas — washed*
*2 Tablespoons fresh lemon juice*

In a wok or skillet, heat oil over medium heat. Add garlic and ginger and sauté for 2 minutes. Add pinenuts, snowpeas, and lemon juice. Sauté about 12-15 minutes. Snowpeas should still be a bit crunchy.

# VEGETABLE CASSEROLE WITH TOFU & SPINACH NOODLES

6-8 servings

1 Tablespoon oil
1 cup onion — chopped
2 garlic cloves — chopped
1/3 cup fresh parsley — chopped
1/2 cup leek — chopped
2 cups eggplant — peeled and chopped into 1-inch cubes
3 Tablespoons fresh basil — chopped
1 cup fresh tomatoes — chopped
1 cup zucchini — sliced thick
1 - 16 ounce can tomatoes — no salt added
1 cup water
1/2 cup bran
Pepper
1 pound plain tofu
1 1/2 cups lowfat mozzarella cheese — grated
1/2 cup parmesan cheese
1 pound spinach lasagna noodles — uncooked

Preheat oven to 350°

Heat oil in a saucepan. Add onion, garlic, parsley, and leek. Cook about 3 minutes. Add eggplant, 1 Tablespoon basil, tomatoes, zucchini, canned tomatoes, water, bran, and pepper. Drain tofu, break into chunks, and place in a bowl with mozzarella, parmesan, 2 Tablespoons basil, and more pepper to taste. Mix well.

Place a little sauce in the bottom of a 9x12 baking dish, then a layer of uncooked spinach lasagna noodles slightly overlapping each other, then a thick layer of tofu-cheese mixture, using about 1/2 of the mixture. Layer sauce, lasagna noodles, cheese mixture, sauce. Bake for 45-50 minutes. Let sit for 10 minutes before cutting.

# CELERIAC WITH MIXED VEGETABLES STIR-FRY

4 servings

*1 Tablespoon olive oil*
*3 Tablespoons leeks — chopped*
*¾ cup red bell pepper — cut into thin strips*
*1 cup celeriac — peel root, cut into 4 and slice thick*
*2 Tablespoons fresh lemon juice*
*1 cup fresh mushrooms — sliced*
*Pepper*

Blanch celeriac 5 minutes in boiling water, drain. In a skillet or wok, heat oil over medium heat. Add leeks and red bell peppers. Sauté a minute or so. Cut blanched celeriac into 1-inch pieces and sprinkle with lemon juice. Add celeriac and mushrooms to skillet. Add pepper to taste. Cook about 3-5 minutes until vegetables are tender but crisp, mixing often.

This dish is very good served with chicken or fish. It's different and refreshing.

# VEGETABLE AND SHRIMP STIR-FRY

4 servings

1 Tablespoon olive oil
3 large garlic cloves — chopped
¼ cup onion — chopped
1 cup yellow squash — sliced thick
½ teaspoon fresh ginger root — grated
¼ cup pineapple juice
½ cup red bell pepper — short strips
¼ cup green onion — chopped
1 - 5¼ ounce can pineapple — drained (save juice)
1 cup shrimp
½ cup bean sprouts — rinsed and drained
½ cup unsalted peanuts — shelled
Pepper

In a skillet or wok, heat oil. Add garlic and onion, and sauté a few minutes. Add squash, ginger, and half of the pineapple juice. Simmer about 3 minutes. Add red bell pepper, green onion, remaining pineapple juice, and pineapple chunks; simmer about 2 minutes. Add shrimp, bean sprouts, peanuts, and pepper. Mix until shrimp are well heated and vegetables are tender.

# YELLOW SPLIT PEA SOUP   Approximately 4 cups

*3 cups water*
*1 cup chicken broth*
*1 Tablespoon Worcestershire sauce*
*1 cup onion — chopped*
*2 garlic cloves — minced*
*¼ cup leeks — chopped*
*½ teaspoon dried thyme*
*1 cup yellow split peas — check for stones and rinse*
*1 Tablespoon fresh parsley — rinsed and chopped*
*¾ cup carrots — quartered and sliced*
*⅓ cup red bell pepper — diced*
*Pepper*

In a saucepan, combine water, chicken broth, Worcestershire sauce, onion, garlic, leeks, and thyme. Bring to a boil. Add split peas and let return to a boil. Lower heat and simmer covered, until peas are slightly tender (about 10 minutes). Add parsley, carrots, and red bell pepper, and simmer, covered, over medium to medium-low heat until peas and carrots are tender (about 20 minutes). Add pepper to taste, if desired.

## WATERCRESS-TURKEY SOUP

4 servings

2 cups water
1 beef bouillon cube
3/4 cup onion — chopped
4 large garlic cloves — chopped
1 cup fresh watercress — chopped
1 cup fresh mushrooms — chopped
1/3 cup fresh parsley — chopped
1 cup carrot — grated
2 cups turkey — chopped
1 1/2 teaspoons dried thyme
1/4 teaspoon poultry seasoning
3 teaspoons Pickapeppa sauce
1 cup water
2 raw chicken wings

In a soup pot, combine 2 cups water, bouillon cube, onion, garlic, and watercress. Simmer until onions are tender. Add mushrooms, parsley, carrot, turkey, thyme, poultry seasoning, Pickapeppa sauce, water, and chicken wings. Simmer 40 minutes-1 hour.

## CREAM OF CORN AND MUSHROOM SOUP

5-6 servings

1 - 14 1/2 ounce can beef broth
1 cup onion — chopped
3 Tablespoons elephant garlic — chopped
1/4 cup leeks — chopped

2½ *cups whole kernel corn — fresh, frozen or canned*
*2 Tablespoons unbleached white flour*
*1 teaspoon unsalted butter*
*1 cup nonfat milk*
*1 cup fresh mushrooms — chopped (optional)*

In a soup pot, combine beef broth, onion, garlic, leeks, and 1½ cups corn. Simmer about 15 minutes on medium heat. Place mixture in a blender and purée (blend half at a time). Set aside. In a pot, combine flour and butter, mixing well. Add milk all at once and stir until mixture starts to thicken. Add corn purée, the remaining cup of corn, and fresh mushrooms (optional). Simmer 10-15 minutes longer on low heat.

# *ACORN SQUASH SOUP*     Approximately 6 cups

*1 - 14¼ ounce can chicken broth*
*3 cups acorn squash — peeled and cubed (2 medium-sized squash)*
*3 cups water*
*1 cup onion — chopped*
¼ *cup leeks — chopped*
*1 teaspoon dried seaweed — crumbled*
*1 cup fresh mushrooms — chopped (optional)*
*Garnish — grated fresh ginger (optional)*

In a soup pan, combine all ingredients, and simmer, uncovered, on medium heat until squash is tender. Place in blender and purée, return to pot, and heat. Serve hot.

# CARROT SOUP

6 servings

*¼ cup leeks — chopped*
*1 - 14½ ounce can chicken broth*
*1 bay leaf*
*2 cups carrots — diced*
*1 teaspoon Pickapeppa sauce*
*2 teaspoons fresh basil — minced*
*2 cups water*
*Pepper*
*1 cup whole kernel corn — fresh, frozen or canned*
*¼ cup red bell pepper — diced*

In a soup pan, combine leeks, broth, bay leaf, carrots, Pickapeppa sauce, basil, water, and pepper. Simmer over medium heat about 5 minutes. Add corn and red bell pepper, continue to simmer until carrots are tender.

# BEAN SOUP

*¼ cup dry kidney beans*
*¼ cup dry garbanzo beans*
*¼ cup dry pink beans*
*¼ cup dry pinto beans*
*1 Tablespoon olive oil*
*½ pound stew meat — browned*
*5 cups water*
*3 garlic cloves — chopped*
*½ cup onion — chopped*
*½ cup chicken broth*
*1 - 9 ounce can tomatoes*
*1½ teaspoons dried oregano*
*2 teaspoons Worcestershire sauce*
*½ cup carrots — julienne cut*
*½ cup celery — julienne cut*
*¼ cup ketchup (optional)*
*Pepper (optional)*
*¼ cup elbow macaroni — cooked and drained*

Wash beans thoroughly, cover with cold water, and soak overnight in refrigerator or a cool place. After soaking, drain beans and rinse with fresh water. In a soup kettle, heat olive oil and brown stew meat. Add water, garlic, beans, and onion. Simmer until beans are tender but firm. Add chicken broth, tomatoes, oregano, Worcestershire sauce, carrots, celery, ketchup, and pepper. Simmer until beef and vegetables are tender, about 15 minutes. Add cooked macaroni, let heat thoroughly, and serve.

# FISH CHOWDER

1 Tablespoon olive oil
1 cup onion — chopped
3/4 cup leeks — chopped
2-3 garlic cloves
1 quart stewed tomatoes
1 - 8 ounce can tomato sauce
1 - 6½ ounce can of chopped clams and juice
½ teaspoon fennel seed
¼ teaspoon dried tarragon
1 teaspoon dried thyme
1 bay leaf
Pepper
1 cup raw potatoes — chopped into 1-inch cubes
½ cup carrots — sliced
½ cup fresh snapper or salmon — cut into large chunks
½ cup fresh asparagus — chopped, about 6 spears
1 cup shrimp

In a soup kettle, heat oil and sauté onions, leeks, and garlic. Add stewed tomatoes, tomato sauce, clams with juice, fennel seed, tarragon, thyme, bay leaf, pepper, potatoes, and carrots. Simmer uncovered for 5 minutes. Rinse and pat dry the fish. Add half the fish and simmer about 10 minutes. Add the rest of the fish, asparagus, and simmer on low until the potatoes are tender, about 10-15 minutes longer. Add shrimp and cook till they are thoroughly heated (about 1 minute).

# CLAM CHOWDER I

Approximately 6 servings

*1 Tablespoon margarine*
*1 cup onion — chopped*
*1 cup celery — chopped*
*¹⁄₄ cup green onion — chopped*
*¹⁄₃ cup red bell pepper — chopped*
*2 - 6¹⁄₂ ounce cans clams — with juice*
*1 - 8 ounce jar clam juice*
*3 Italian tomatoes*
*¹⁄₂ cup tomato sauce*
*1 - 14 ounce can tomatoes*
*2¹⁄₂ teaspoons dried thyme*
*1 teaspoon ground cumin*
*1 cup corn — fresh, frozen, or canned*

In a saucepan, melt margarine. Add onion, celery, and green onion, and sauté for a few minutes. Add red bell pepper, clams and clam juice, Italian tomatoes, tomato sauce, canned tomatoes, thyme, cumin, and corn. Let simmer on low heat 25-35 minutes.

# CLAM CHOWDER II

½ cup nitrate-free bacon — chopped
¾ cup onion — diced
¾ cup celery — diced
1½ Tablespoons fresh parsley — chopped
1 Tablespoon margarine
2 cups fresh clams — or 2 cans clams (5-8 ounces) with juice
1 bay leaf
2 cups clam juice — or 1 - 8 ounce jar clam juice
1½ teaspoons dried thyme
2 teaspoons dried basil
2 Tablespoons canned pimientos — drained and chopped
¼ teaspoon onion salt — optional
2 cups potatoes — peeled and diced
2 cups 2% milk
3 Tablespoons unbleached white flour
⅓ cup water

In a large saucepan, fry bacon until crisp, then drain. Add onion, celery, and fresh parsley and sauté until celery is tender. Add margarine. Sauté about 2 more minutes. Add clams (if using canned clams, use juice), bay leaf, clam juice, thyme, basil, pimiento, onion salt, potatoes, and milk. Mix well. Simmer uncovered on medium heat, stirring often, for 35-40 minutes.
Combine flour and ⅓ cup water, and add to soup, stirring constantly. Let simmer about 5 more minutes and serve.

If by chance you put too much salt in soup, stew, or chili, you can cut a raw potato into a few pieces and add them to the broth. The potato pieces will draw out the salt. Remove potato before serving.

# POTATO SOUP

*½ cup nitrate-free raw bacon — chopped*
*1 cup onion — chopped*
*¾ cup celery — chopped*
*1 Tablespoon margarine*
*3 cups water*
*¼ cup flour*
*3 cups raw potatoes — diced into 1-inch cubes*
*Pinch of salt — optional*
*White pepper*
*1 teaspoon Worcestershire sauce*
*½ cup 2% milk*
*1 Tablespoon fresh parsley — chopped*

In a skillet, fry bacon and drain off excess grease. Add onion, celery, and margarine. Sauté until celery is tender. In a soup kettle, combine sautéed bacon mixture, pre-mixed flour and water, potatoes, salt, pepper, and Worcestershire sauce. Simmer, covered, over medium-low heat about 30-45 minutes, or until potatoes are tender. Add milk and parsley, mix well, and continue to cook until thoroughly heated.

Note: ⅓ cup carrots (grated) an optional addition. Garnish with fresh chopped tomato, if desired.

## CREAM OF CARROT SOUP  Approximately 6 cups

2 cups carrots — chopped
2 cups water
1 cup fresh mushrooms — sliced
1 cup onion — chopped
1 Tablespoon margarine
1 bay leaf
Pepper
1 cup Brussels sprouts — washed, halved, and steamed until tender
1½ cups 2% or nonfat milk

In a large saucepan, combine carrots, water, mushrooms, onion, margarine, bay leaf, and pepper. Simmer until carrots are tender. Remove bay leaf. Place carrot mixture in blender and purée lightly. Return to saucepan. Add steamed Brussels sprouts and milk. Heat thoroughly and serve.

## SANDY'S SPLIT PEA SOUP  Approximately 6 cups

5 cups water
²/₃ cup onion — diced
²/₃ cup celery — diced (use leaves as well as rib)
3 garlic cloves — pressed
2 Tablespoons low-sodium soy sauce
3 Tablespoons sherry (California Golden)
1¾ cups green split peas — rinse and check for rocks
1 cup carrots — shredded
Salt and pepper to taste

In a soup pan, combine water, onion, celery, garlic, soy sauce, and

**164**

sherry. Bring to a boil, lower heat, and simmer until onions and celery are tender. Add split peas, carrots, and salt and pepper (if desired). Bring to boil, lower heat to medium or medium-low. Simmer, covered, until peas are tender but not mushy, 45 minutes-1 hour.

---

## RUTABAGA-TURNIP SOUP Approximately 6 cups

*1 pound lean stew meat — cubed*
*2 Tablespoons olive oil*
*$1/2$ cup onion — chopped*
*1 garlic clove — diced*
*$3/4$ cup green bell pepper — diced*
*$1/2$ cup celery — diced*
*1 - 14 ounce can of tomatoes*
*2 shots Tabasco (more if desired)*
*$1^1/2$ cups water*
*$1/4$ cup ketchup*
*Dash of salt — optional*
*Pepper*
*1 cup carrots — chopped*
*1 cup potatoes — chopped*
*1 cup rutabaga — chopped*
*1 cup turnips — chopped*
*Another $1^1/2$ cups water*

In a soup pan, brown stew meat in olive oil. Add onion, garlic, and green bell pepper, and sauté for a few minutes. Add celery, tomatoes, Tabasco, $1^1/2$ cups water, ketchup, salt, and pepper. Simmer over medium-low heat for 1 hour. Add carrots, potatoes, rutabagas, turnips, $1^1/2$ cups water, and more pepper to taste. Simmer, covered, over medium-low heat until vegetables are done. Add more water if necessary, and more ketchup if desired.

# THICK BROCCOLI SOUP         Approximately 6 cups

2 cups chicken broth
1 cup onion — chopped
½ teaspoon dried marjoram
2 teaspoons garlic — chopped
3 cups fresh broccoli — chopped
1 cup peeled potatoes — diced
1 teaspoon dried thyme
1 bay leaf
1 Tablespoon margarine
2 Tablespoons flour
¼ teaspoon white pepper — optional
2 cups 2% milk

In a large saucepan, combine chicken broth, onion, marjoram, garlic, broccoli, potatoes, thyme, and bay leaf. Bring to a boil and simmer until broccoli is tender. Remove from heat, take out bay leaf and discard. Purée broccoli mixture in blender (half at a time) until smooth. Set aside. In a soup pan, melt margarine. Blend in flour and pepper. Add 1 cup of milk all at once, stirring over medium heat until mixture thickens. Stir in broccoli purée and remaining cup of milk. Mix well. Cook until thoroughly heated.

# CHICKEN SOUP MANDY'S WAY 4 servings

If using a larger or smaller chicken than the recipe uses, be sure to adjust water a bit.

*1 - 2 or 2½ pound chicken*
*4½-5 cups water*
*5 garlic cloves — chopped*
*1 cup onion — chopped*
*¾-1 cup green bell pepper — chopped*
*1 cup celery — chopped*
*4 fresh tomatoes — chopped (15 ounce can of tomatoes may be used)*
*Salt and pepper to taste — optional*
*2 Tablespoons rice — raw (use white, brown or basmati)*
*¾ cup zucchini or yellow squash — sliced*
*Optional for garnish: sour cream and avocado*

Wash chicken and remove as much of the skin as you can. In a soup pan, combine water and chicken. Cook about 30-40 minutes, or until chicken is tender. Remove the chicken from pan, take the meat off the bones, and return meat to pan. Add garlic, onion, green bell pepper, celery, tomatoes, and desired amount of salt and pepper. Simmer for 30 minutes. Add rice and simmer for 15 minutes. Add zucchini (or yellow squash) and simmer for another 10 minutes. Garnish if desired.

# CREAM OF BRUSSELS SPROUTS AND MUSHROOM SOUP

8 cups

*2 cups chicken broth*
*1 cup onion — chopped*
*1 cup fresh mushrooms — chopped*
*3 cups fresh Brussels sprouts — washed and quartered (frozen can be used)*
*¼ cup California golden sherry*
*1 teaspoon dried basil*
*1 teaspoon dried thyme*
*3 Tablespoons raw nitrate-free bacon — chopped*
*1 teaspoon margarine*
*2 Tablespoons unbleached white flour*
*2 cups 2% milk*
*White pepper — optional*

In a large saucepan, combine chicken broth, onions, mushrooms, Brussels sprouts, sherry, basil, and thyme. Bring to a boil, reduce heat and simmer, covered, until Brussels sprouts are tender (about 10-12 minutes). Remove from heat and place ⅔ of mixture in a blender, purée until smooth, return to pan with remaining ⅓ of mixture and set aside. In another saucepan, cook bacon until done, drain off excess grease (if any), and heat margarine. Add flour and mix well. Add 1 cup milk all at once and stir over medium heat until mixture boils and thickens. Add Brussels sprouts mixture, remaining cup of milk, and pepper. Stir well. Continue cooking until thoroughly heated.

# TASTY TURKEY SOUP

6-8 servings

Make after a turkey meal.

*Turkey carcass and turkey scraps*
*2 bay leaves*
*1 cup onion — chopped*
*Pepper*
*Water*
*½ cup brown rice — raw*
*1 cup carrots — julienne cut*
*1 cup zucchini (with skin) — chopped*
*2 ears of corn — broken into small pieces (about 6)*
*1 teaspoon dried rosemary — crushed*
*1 cup turkey meat — cut into 1-inch pieces or larger*
*½ teaspoon flax seed*
*Salt — optional*

In a soup kettle, combine carcass, turkey scraps, bay leaves, onion, pepper, and water to cover. Simmer, covered, 1 hour. Remove carcass and strain broth. Return strained broth to kettle and add brown rice. Bring to a boil, lower heat, and add carrots, zucchini, corn, rosemary, turkey meat, and flax seed. Cook, covered, until vegetables are tender. Let sit a few minutes before serving.

Note: Flax seed will thicken soup. May substitute 3 Tablespoons flour and ¼ cup water. Mix well and stir into soup.

# NOODLE SOUP

4 servings

*3 cups water*
*1 cup potatoes — sliced thin*
*¼ teaspoon garlic powder*
*Pepper — to taste*
*2 cups uncooked fresh egg noodles — buy at market or see pasta*
*    recipes on pages 282-284*
*1 Tablespoon olive oil*

In a soup pan, combine 3 cups water, potatoes, garlic powder, and pepper. Bring to a boil and cook, covered, 5 minutes. Add 1 cup egg noodles, lower heat, and simmer. Meanwhile, in a skillet, heat olive oil and add 1 cup egg noodles. Cook until browned evenly. Add browned noodles to potato/noodle mixture. Mix well. Simmer until noodles are done. Serve hot.

# BORSCHT

*1¹/₂-2 pounds short ribs*
*6 cups water*
*1 cup onion — cut into large pieces*
*1 Tablespoon pickling spice (remove garlic and cinnamon)*
*Pepper to taste*
*2 cups beets — boiled in water 20 minutes, drained, and cubed*
*2 cups onions — chopped*
*2 cups potatoes — diced*
*1 - 16 ounce can tomatoes*
*2 to 3 beef bouillon cubes dissolved in ¹/₄ cup water*
*2 cups water*
*2 cups cabbage — shredded*

In a large soup pan, combine ribs, water, 1 cup onion, pickling spice, and pepper. Boil for 30 minutes, then simmer, covered, for 1¹/₂ hours or until beef is tender. Remove beef and strip meat from bones. Cut into small pieces and place back into kettle. Add beets, 2 cups onions, potatoes, tomatoes, and bouillon. Add 2 cups water or enough to cover. Simmer until potatoes are almost tender. Add the cabbage and simmer until potatoes are done.

Note: Rice, barley, or tomato juice may be added if desired. Borscht is even better the next day.
Sour cream is sometimes used as a garnish.

# PIZZA

Pizza has a bad reputation as a junk food full of calories, cholesterol, and fat. But pizza is really a very good source of protein, complex carbohydrates, vitamins, minerals, and fiber. Without the sausage, pepperoni, and bacon, pizza is lower in fat than you may think. Of course, pizzas vary a great deal in nutritional content depending on what you use to build them with. Meat toppings and high cheese content raise the fat and cholesterol levels. Vegetables will boost vitamin and fiber content. Add a whole wheat or cornmeal crust for extra fiber and extra flavor. For whole wheat crust, see whole wheat bread recipe on page 256. Or try your own favorite bread recipe. If time is short, use either a package of hot roll mix or uncooked frozen bread dough.

## PIZZA SAUCE
*1 Tablespoon olive oil*
*3-4 large garlic cloves — pressed or chopped*
*²/₃ cup onion — chopped*
*2 Tablespoons fresh parsley — chopped*
*½ cup mushrooms — sliced*
*¼ cup green pepper — diced*
*½ teaspoon dried thyme*
*½ teaspoon dried green oregano*
*1 teaspoon dried basil*
*⅓ cup water*
*1 - 9 ounce can tomatoes*
*2 - 8 ounce cans tomato sauce*

In a saucepan, heat oil. Add garlic, onions, and parsley, and sauté 2-3 minutes. Add remaining ingredients and simmer on low-medium heat until sauce thickens, about 45 minutes. Makes enough for two pizzas. Eat one and freeze one.

172

Spread sauce over crust. Add toppings and bake at 350° for 15-20 minutes. If making individual small pizzas, bake about 10-12 minutes.

WHAT? You can't think of any toppings? Choose from a few of our favorites.
Anchovies — drained
Black olives
Mushrooms
Lowfat swiss cheese
2% mozzarella cheese
Onions
Green onions
Red bell peppers
Green bell peppers
Shrimp
Salmon — cooked
Broccoli
Tomatoes
Marinated artichoke hearts

Pizzas are fun at parties. Make small individual crusts and let everyone create their own.
Also check other sauces on pages 141, 142, 147, and 149.

# NOTES

# NOTES

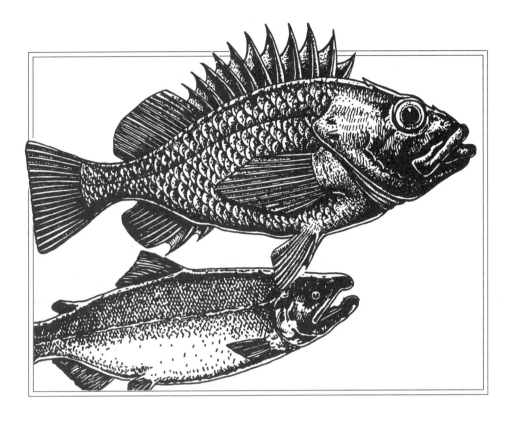

# SEAFOOD

# SEVEN STEPS TO A HEALTHIER HEART

1. Stop smoking cigarettes.

2. Exercise regularly.

3. Reduce fats and cholesterol in the diet.

4. Control high blood pressure.

5. Check with your doctor before using oral contraceptive pills.

6. Get tested regularly for diabetes.

7. Get regular medical check-ups.

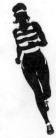

# *FISH*

Fish is an excellent source of minerals, including iodine, magnesium, calcium, phosphorus, iron, potassium, copper, and fluoride. Some fatty fish are high in vitamin D. Swordfish and white fish are high in vitamin A. The protein in fish is of very high quality, and provides a generous amount and variety of the amino acids the body needs. This protein is more easily digested than that of chicken or meat.

The American Institute of Cancer Research, along with many other experts, believes that fish oil, with its high-quality polyunsaturated oil known as omega 3 fatty acid, may alleviate high blood pressure and reduce chances of heart and blood vessel diseases; it may play an important role in protection against breast and prostate cancers; and may also help inflammation in cases of arthritis and asthma. (See pages 26-32 on Fat and Cholesterol for more information.)

Fish is also generally low in sodium and, contrary to popular belief, saltwater fish have no higher sodium content than freshwater fish. If you are concerned with sodium content, avoid all smoked fish and salt-cured fish. Because fish contains little or no connective tissue, it is very easy to digest and is suitable for all diets. Remember, fish is great for breakfast, lunch, or dinner.

## HOW TO CHOOSE A FRESH FISH

Buy the freshest fish you can get.

• Fish should not have a discernible odor, and certainly not a "fishy smell."

• Eyes should be clear and bulging: The fresher the fish, the clearer, shinier, and brighter the eyes. If the fish is aging, the eyes become sunken and increasingly cloudy.

• Skin should be shiny and bright, and scales tight and firm to touch. In addition the film covering the skin should be clear, not cloudy.

• Fresh gills are a nice reddish color and have a clean smell. When a fish begins to deteriorate, the gills are the first parts to go. The color changes from reddish to a dark brown or gray and the fish begins giving off a "fishy" or foul odor.

Remember, if you buy an old fish you won't be able to disguise the "off" taste.

Shellfish also must be very fresh. Seafood such as lobsters, clams, crabs, oysters, and mussels should be purchased live. Because of the possibility of bacterial infections, fresh fish and shellfish should not remain at room temperature for more than two hours. They should be refrigerated at 35-40° in a leakproof wrapper. Use as soon as possible after purchasing, but cook within two days for sure. Frozen fish and shellfish should not be thawed at room temperature. They should be thawed slowly in the refrigerator (still in their wrappings). Never refrigerate thawed fish or shellfish longer than 24 hours before cooking. (See pages 44-47 on Food Safety, for more information.)

The main rule for fine fish cooking is DO NOT OVERCOOK. Fish cooks quickly. Overcooking robs it of its juices and produces a dry and flabby texture. One rule for cooking fish is to allow 10 minutes per inch of thickness. (To determine thickness, measure thickest part of fish with a ruler.) The 10-minute rule applies for all cooking methods except microwaving. Fish is cooked when the flesh becomes opaque and flakes easily with a fork. Poaching, steaming, baking, broiling, microwaving, and stir-frying are excellent lowfat cooking methods. Select any of these methods to keep the calorie and fat content of your seafood dishes low.

| LEAN FISH | MODERATELY FATTY FISH | FATTY FISH |
|---|---|---|
| Black Bass | Albacore | Anchovies |
| Bluefish | Bluefin Tuna | Bluefish |
| Bonita | Bonita | Bonita |
| Brook Trout | Carp | Butterfish |
| Bullhead | Chum Salmon | Chinook Salmon |
| Catfish | Dolly Varden Trout | Dogfish |
| Cod | Mullet | Eel |
| Crappie | Pink Salmon | Herring |
| Croaker | Porgy | Jack Mackerel |
| Flounder | Rainbow Trout | Mackerel |
| Grouper | Sablefish | Most Trout |
| Haddock | Sea Trout | Mullet |
| Hake | Sole | Pompano |
| Halibut | Sturgeon | Sablefish |
| Lingcod | Swordfish | Sardines |
| Ocean Perch | | Shad |
| Pike | | Sockeye Salmon |
| Pollock | | Spot |
| Rockfish | | Steelhead |
| Sea Bass | | Tuna (unless |
| Shark | | canned in |
| Smelt | | water) |
| Snapper | | Whitefish |
| Spotted Sea Trout | | |
| Sunfish | | |
| Tilefish | | |
| Walleye | | |
| White Seabass | | |
| Whiting | | |
| Yellow Perch | | |
| Yellowfin Tuna | | |

## Analysis Based on 50% Leg Meat and 50% Body Meat

| 100 GRAM PORTIONS | PROTEIN | FAT | CARBOHYDRATE | CALORIES | SODIUM |
|---|---|---|---|---|---|
| King Crab | 18.0 | 2.0 | 0.0 | 95.0 | 100.0-900.0* |
| Dungeness Crab | 19.4 | 0.9 | 0.0 | 91.0 | 900.0 |
| Snow Crab | 18.8 | 1.3 | 0.0 | 91.6 | |
| Shrimp | 18.1 | 1.0 | 0.0 | 86.0 | 480.0 |
| Salmon | | | | | |
|   King (Chinook) | 20.0 | 12.0 | 0.0 | 188.0 | |
|   Sockeye (Red) | 20.0 | 9.0 | 0.0 | 161.0 | |
|   Silver (Coho) | 22.0 | 5.0 | 0.0 | 133.0 | |
|   Pink | 19.0 | 5.0 | 0.0 | 121.0 | |
|   Chum | 21.0 | 4.0 | 0.0 | 120.0 | |
| Halibut | 21.2 | 0.7 | 0.0 | 97.0 | 53.0 |
| Cod | 17.2 | 0.7 | 0.0 | 79.0 | 70.3 |
| Sablefish | 12.9 | 15.2 | 0.0 | 192.0 | 56.0 |
| Rockfish | 19.0 | 1.5 | 0.0 | 95.5 | 63.0 |
| Pollock | 17.5 | 0.9 | 0.0 | 78.0 | 70.0 |

*Depends on process used in preparing crab.

Source: Alaska Seafood Marketing Institute. Compilation and review data by John A. Dassow, Deputy Director (ret.) & Jerry K. Babbit, Supervisory Food Technologist, Northwest & Alaska Fisheries Center, NOAA, Seattle, Washington, U.S. Dept. of Commerce, Utilization Research Division.

# SALMON

Throughout the ages, the salmon has been held in the highest esteem. Today, the best and largest supply of salmon comes from the icy waters of Alaska. Few single foods bring as many valuable contributions to the table in such significant quantities as does the Alaskan salmon. It is an excellent source of high-quality protein, containing all of the essential amino acids. Salmon contains vitamins A and D, as well as niacin and riboflavin from the B-complex group. Iron, magnesium, and phosphorus are also present in appreciable amounts. The fats in salmon are predominantly unsaturated. There is evidence to indicate these unsaturated fats help avoid development of artery disease (atherosclerosis).

Much of this Alaskan salmon is canned, but there is still an ample year-round supply of fresh-frozen salmon, thanks to modern processing methods, freezing, and transportation. Alaskan salmon can also be found smoked, salted, and kippered.

**King** (Chinook) — It is the largest of the salmon, averaging 11-30 pounds in size, but has been known to reach 125 pounds. King salmon is generally marketed as fillets, steaks, roasts, or whole dressed. The species begins running in the spring and is caught throughout Alaskan waters. King salmon is generally the variety that is smoked, because of its rich oil content.

**Sockeye** (Red or Blue) — The Sockeye averages about 6 pounds. Deep red in color and rich in oil, sockeye salmon is primarily marketed in cans. The remainder is available fresh or frozen.

**Pink** — Smallest of all the salmon, Pinks average 2-5 pounds in weight. They are the most plentiful of all the species and range in color from light to deep pink. Pink salmon is primarily marketed in cans but is also available fresh or frozen in season.

**Silver** (Coho) — Averaging 4-12 pounds, silvers are generally marketed fresh or frozen in steaks or fillets.

**Chum** (Silver Brite) — Chum averages about 7 pounds, is lighter in color and has less oil than other varieties. Chum is primarily caught in August and September.

*Source: Alaska Seafood Marketing Institute*

# HOW TO FILLET A WHOLE SALMON

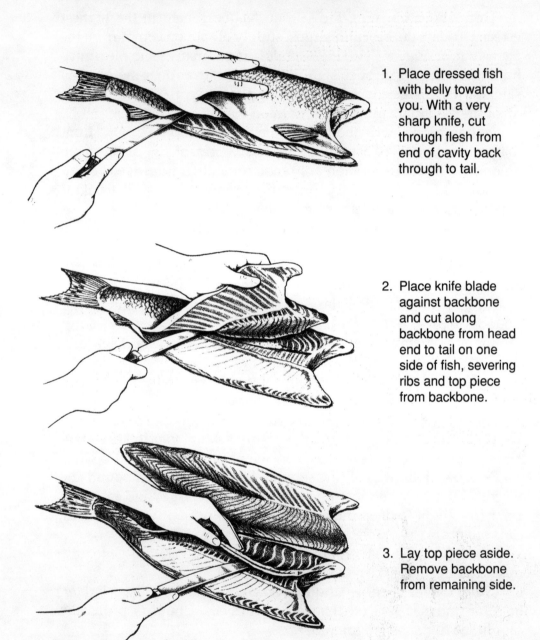

1. Place dressed fish with belly toward you. With a very sharp knife, cut through flesh from end of cavity back through to tail.

2. Place knife blade against backbone and cut along backbone from head end to tail on one side of fish, severing ribs and top piece from backbone.

3. Lay top piece aside. Remove backbone from remaining side.

184

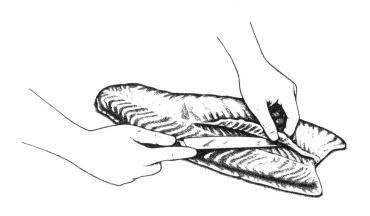

4. With a smaller knife, trim away rib and fin bones from both pieces. Pull out pin bones, if desired.

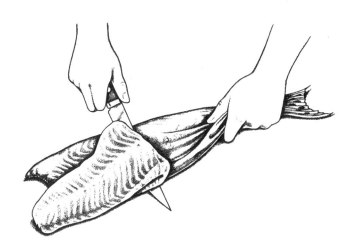

5. If you wish to skin fillets, place skin-side-down on cutting surface. Hold tail end tightly. With sharp knife, cut down through the flesh to skin. Flatten knife against skin and cut flesh away by sliding it toward head end while holding tail end of skin firmly.

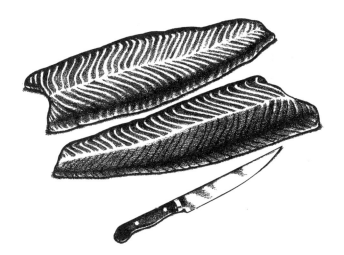

6. Prepared salmon fillets can be baked, poached or grilled, or cut into serving-sized portions.

185

## COOKING METHODS

*Baked* — Place in well-greased or foil-lined baking dish. Brush fish with melted margarine, lemon, or favorite sauce. Bake at 350°, allowing 10 minutes per inch of thickness measured at its thickest part. Stuff dressed salmon if desired and measure thickness after stuffing. Do not turn fish during baking.

*Broil* — Place salmon steaks or fillets on a well-greased broiler pan. Brush fish with olive oil or favorite sauce. Place in oven 4 inches from broiler. Broil 10 minutes per inch of thickness measured at thickest part. Turn salmon halfway through cooking time, brush with oil or sauce, continue cooking until salmon flakes when tested with fork at thickest part.

*Grill* — Place salmon on hot grill. Allow 10 minutes per inch, measured at thickest part. Turn once. Baste salmon with oil or favorite sauce. Salmon is done when flaky at thickest part. See barbecued salmon recipe on page 206.

*Sauté* — Place in a heated skillet with olive oil. Sauté salmon, covered, until done. Cooking time will be approximately 10 minutes per inch of thickness measured at its thickest part.

*Microwave* — Place 1 salmon steak (about 6 ounces) in microwave-proof dish; cover dish with plastic wrap. Microwave at medium $1^{1}/_{2}$-2 minutes; rotate dish one quarter turn halfway through cooking time. Drain juices, cover tightly with wrap. Let stand 5 minutes.

## HOW TO CAN SALMON

Only fresh fish should be canned, and should be bled and thoroughly cleaned when caught or as soon afterwards as possible.

- Draw fish (remove entrails). Remove scales, fins, and head. Clean and wash with fresh water. Can with skin on.
- Cut fish into large pieces (leave backbone in unless it is too large for cans).
- Soak fish in brine ($^{1}/_{4}$-$^{1}/_{2}$ cup salt to 1 gallon water) to draw out blood for 30-60 minutes depending on thickness of fish. If fish is soft, soak for 1-2 hours in the brine.

- Pre-heat clean cans or jars by setting them into boiling water until steaming hot.
- Drain well before packing. Pack pieces skin side out, add no water or salt, and pack to within 1 inch from top. Put on cap and screw band FIRMLY TIGHT. If using cans, seal accordingly.
- PROCESS: Pint jars 100 minutes at 10 pounds pressure.
  Quart jars 100 minutes at 10 pounds pressure.
  Number two cans 90 minutes at 10 pounds pressure.
  Larger containers are not recommended for fish.
- Remove cans or jars from pressure cooker, seal or check seal according to type of container used, cool in tepid water. Store glass containers in dark dry place.

Note: Halibut is improved by the addition of 1 teaspoon of olive oil to each can.

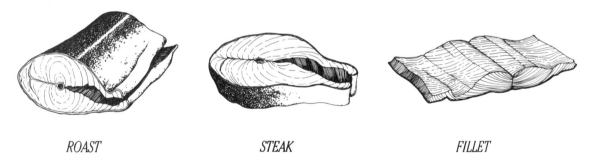

ROAST             STEAK             FILLET

# POACHING

Poaching is a low calorie, flavorful, and efficient cooking method that can be used with almost any fish, cut or whole, with the exception of those that are excessively small (smelt, herring), fibrous (marlin), or oily (mackerel). Poaching is especially good with salmon or a delicate fish like sole. Contrary to popular opinion, poaching is not "boiling." Instead, it is a gentle process where fish is submerged in a flavored liquid and barely simmered to perfection. If you have a fresh fish, a shallow pan or skillet, water, herbs or fresh lemon juice, and 15-20 minutes, you can be a poaching success.

**First:**  Choose your poaching liquid.
- 2 cups water/2 Tablespoons vinegar
- Water and wine 50/50
- chicken stock
- milk, or water with any combination of herbs, lemon juice, or seaweeds

Salmon is delicious with celery or clam base added to the water. Let poaching liquid simmer for 10-15 minutes, and you're ready to go. Poaching liquids can be made up ahead of time and frozen.

**Second:** When you're ready to cook, bring the liquid to a simmer in a broad, shallow pan. Gently slip fish into the liquid, adding water necessary to cover completely. Simmer on low heat, covered, allowing 10 minutes per inch of thickness. Once cooked, remove the fish carefully with a spatula in both hands. Freshly poached fish is very fragile and tricky to handle. When poaching a whole fish, it is wise to wrap the fish in a layer or two of cheesecloth, leaving it a bit long, like a handle, on each end of the fish. This makes removing the fish easier, and prevents it from falling apart.

Remember that chilled poached fish is excellent for brunch, salads, or lunch.

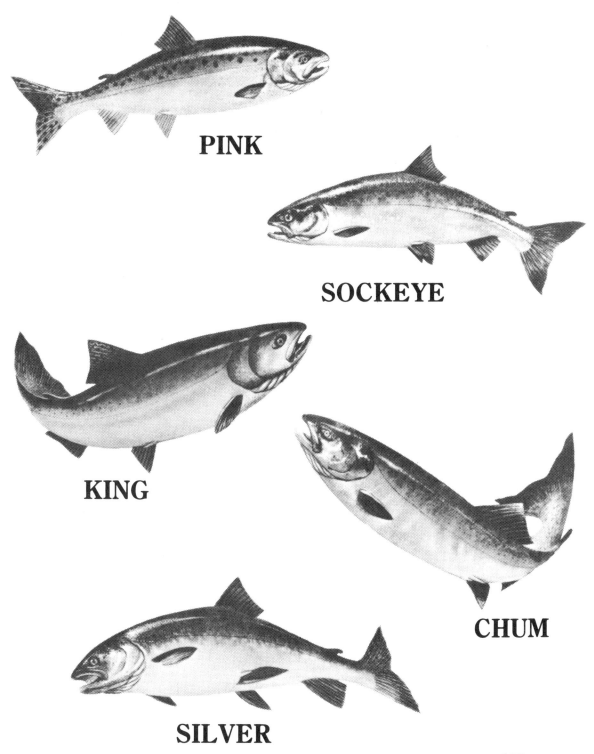

**PINK**

**SOCKEYE**

**KING**

**CHUM**

**SILVER**

189

# CRAB

**King Crab** — Alaskan King crab is one of the largest members of the entire crab family, which includes more than 1,000 species. The largest King crab ever caught weighed 25 pounds and measured 6 feet from claw to claw. King crab is easily recognized by its large pieces of succulent white meat, brilliantly edged in red. King crab is prized for its delicate flavor, tender texture, and convenience. It is an excellent source of high-quality protein, containing all of the essential amino acids, and is low in fat and calories. King crab also contains important minerals such as zinc, iodine, copper, magnesium, and iron. King crab is marketed year round, in whole or split legs and claws, as well as frozen meat already extracted from the shell.

**Dungeness Crab** — Dungeness crab is a versatile delicacy widely found throughout Alaska's icy waters. This succulent crab has a distinctive, almost sweet flavor, and tender, flaky white meat. Dungeness crab is marketed year round in several forms and, like other varieties of crab, is an excellent source of high-quality protein, containing all essential amino acids, while being low in fat. Important minerals present: iodine, copper, zinc, phosphorus, calcium, magnesium, and iron.

**Snow Crab** — Snow crab is noted for its sweet, delicate flavor and snowy white meat. Snow crab is light in calories, low in fat and is an excellent source of high-quality protein. Snow crab contains copper, zinc, iodine and iron.

## PURCHASE

King — When purchasing King crab legs to serve as an entrée, allow 5-6 ounces per serving. When purchasing King crab meat that has been removed from the shell, allow 2-3 ounces per serving.

Dungeness — One whole 2-3 pound Alaska Dungeness crab will yield about 10 ounces or about 2 cups crab meat. Allow about 2-3 ounces crab meat for each serving.

Snow — When purchasing whole Alaska Snow crab, allow 6-8 ounces for each main dish serving.

*STORAGE*

Alaska King crab and Alaska Snow crab, cleaned and properly wrapped, can be stored in the home freezer at 0° F or lower up to 4 months.

Alaska Dungeness crab in the shell may be stored, properly wrapped, in the home freezer at 0° F or lower up to 10 months. For optimum quality, thawed crab or crab meat can be stored in refrigerator for 1-2 days.

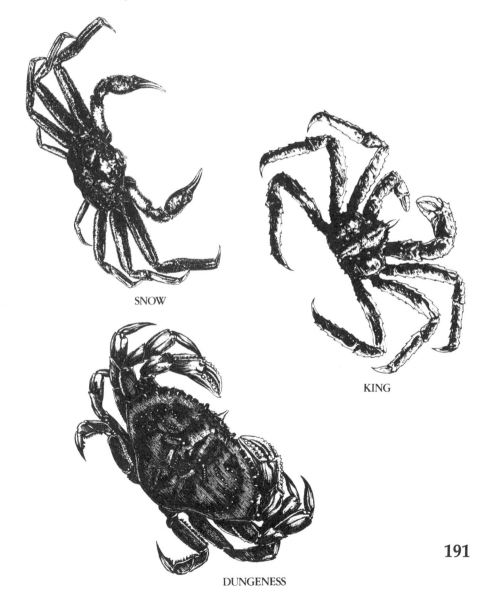

SNOW

KING

DUNGENESS

# CLEANING, CRACKING, AND REMOVING CRAB MEAT

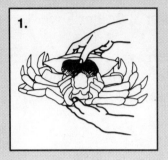

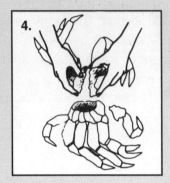

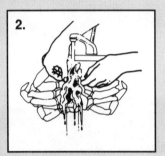

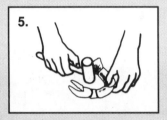

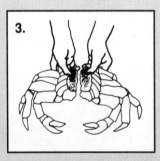

1. If necessary, thaw crab according to thawing directions. Remove broad back shell by holding base of crab with one hand while placing thumb of other hand under shell at mid-point and lifting off back.

2. Remove and discard viscera (the semi-liquid material remaining in the body cavity — it is not normally eaten) and feathery gills from body section. Rinse crab thoroughly under cool, running water, washing away all loose material.

3. Grasp crab in both hands and break in half, yielding two sections with legs attached.

4. Separate legs from each other, one at a time, leaving a portion of body attached to each leg for easy handling.

5. Crack the shell of each claw/leg/body section at edge of joints with small meat mallet to loosen shell; break to expose meat. Meat can then be removed with top of leg, small pick or fork.

## COOKING METHODS

*Thaw* — Place crab in a shallow pan, cover with plastic wrap or foil, and thaw in refrigerator 8-10 hours or overnight. Crab can be thawed in the microwave oven according to manufacturer's directions. In general, one whole 2-3 pound crab may be thawed at defrost, or 30% power, about 20 minutes, covered with waxed paper. Turn crab over and microwave 20 minutes longer. Allow to stand 20 minutes.

*Steam* — Place steamer basket in a large pot. Fill pot with boiling water to approximately $^3/_4$ inch depth. Place crab in basket, reduce heat and steam, covered, about 5 minutes or until crab is thoroughly heated.

*Sauté* — Add crab to heated margarine or oil in pan and sauté 3-5 minutes or until thoroughly heated. When preparing your favorite recipe, add crab during the last 5 minutes of cooking.

*Simmer* — Add crab to soups and stews during the last 5 minutes.

*Broil* — Place crab on broiler rack 5 inches from heat. Broil about 5 minutes or until thoroughly heated. Place King crab split legs in broiler pan, shell side down. Brush with butter or favorite sauce. Place pan about 4 inches from heat. Broil 3-4 minutes. Brush occasionally with butter or sauce while broiling.

*Grill* — Place crab on rack 5 inches above hot coals. Grill about 5 minutes or until thoroughly heated. Place King crab legs or split legs on grill, shell side down. Grill about 5 minutes, brushing with sauce or butter.

*Microwave* — In microwave-proof dish, microwave crab according to oven manufacturer's directions. In general, 1 pound crab, heated at medium, takes about 2-4 minutes.

# SHRIMP

The Alaskan pink shrimp, also referred to as northern shrimp or salad shrimp, is a tiny crustacean harvested throughout the icy waters of Alaska.

These quality shrimp are prized for their convenience. They are completely cooked and peeled during processing. Pink shrimp are lean and tender, with a delicate sweetness. They are also an excellent source of high-quality protein, containing all the essential amino acids, with iodine, zinc, copper, phosphorus, calcium, magnesium, and iron also present. Marketed year round, these shrimp can be found either in the seafood or canned goods section of your supermarket. Because they are already cooked, they are easily incorporated into a wide variety of recipes, heated or chilled. They take well to many seasonings, are delicious in appetizers, salads, stir-fry, soups, casseroles, sauces, and microwave dishes.

*Purchase* — One pound of thawed shrimp will yield 3½ cups. Allow about 3 ounces of shrimp per serving. One cup of loosely packed shrimp weighs about 5 ounces.

*Storage* — May be stored, properly wrapped in freezer at 0° F or lower, up to three months; in refrigerator, about one day.

*Thaw* — Refrigerate 6-7 hours or overnight, or in microwave according to manufacturer's directions.

*Heat* — Since they are already cooked, add to recipes during last 5 minutes of cooking to prevent overcooking and toughness.

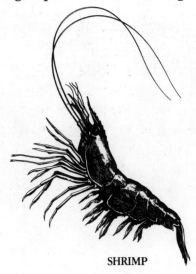

**194**

SHRIMP

# CLAMS

Clams are an extremely healthy food when eaten raw, but they must be fresh. They are rich in mineral salts, especially calcium, potassium, iron, and phosphorus. Cooking destroys some of these minerals and much of the vitamin content, yet clams are still unusually nutritious. Lack of freshness is the chief hazard in buying clams. Only those whose shells are tightly closed are unmistakably fresh. See page 180 for more information on storing and thawing clams.

| CLAMS 3 oz. = 85 gm | protein (g.) | fat (g.) | sat. fat (g.) | calcium (mg.) | phosphorus (mg.) | iron (mg.) | potassium (mg.) | vit. A Intl. units |
|---|---|---|---|---|---|---|---|---|
| RAW | 11 | 1 | 0 | 59 | 138 | 5.2 | 154 | 90 |
| CANNED | 7 | 1 | 0.2 | 47 | 116 | 3.5 | 119 | 0 |

**Butter Clams** — These clams are a West Coast delicacy. The smooth shells are etched with circular growth lines. The small clams are more tender than the large ones. During low tide, dig down about 10-12 inches in gravel-mud areas. All butter clam meat can be eaten raw, steamed, baked, or broiled.

**Donax Clams** — These clams have pink, blue, white, or yellow shells and are found in profusion on sandy beaches from Long Island to the Gulf of Mexico. Usually used for broth.

**Gaper Clams** (Summer Clams, Horse Clams, Blue Clams) — The gaper is found on the Atlantic Coast of the United States, buried in the sand at low water. It favors the mouths of rivers and estuaries. Gapers have large shells, 6-8 inches in size, that gape at either end, and sometimes weigh up to 4 pounds. They lie 2-3 feet under the surface. When gapers are steamed, the body meat is tender, but the neck needs to be pounded before cooking to tenderize.

**Geoduck Clams** — Largest clams on the West Coast shores,

found from Northern California to Alaska, they can weigh up to 6 or 7 pounds, but the average size is about 3 pounds. Shells are white and marked with growth lines. Like the gaper clam, the geoduck is so large the shell cannot close. Geoducks live 2-4 feet below the surface, and are best gathered during the extraordinarily low spring tides. A 3-pound geoduck will yield about 1 pound of meat. Can be purchased fresh or frozen.

**Pismo Clams** — Once very plentiful, these clams are now so depleted that in order to gather them legally, they must measure at least 5 inches across. Pismo clams are large and triangular, with heavy, smooth, polished white shells. They live just below the low-tide line of wave-pounded beaches. They are found in great numbers only in Baja California.

**Quahog Clams** — A popular Atlantic Coast clam, in season year round. Quahogs have heart-shaped, thick, dirty gray/white shells. The quahog clam has a creamy white interior with purple patches. Quahogs bigger than $3^1/_2$ inches are not eaten raw, but usually ground up for chowder.

**Razor Clams** — Fragile, thin, sharp, brownish shells that resemble an old-fashioned straight razor in a folded position. Found in fine-grained sandy beaches. Plentiful in Alaska, British Columbia, Oregon, and Washington. Sold fresh in the Northwest, but also available canned and frozen. Delicious sautéed and in stews.

**Soft-Shell Clams** (Long-neck or Steamer Clams) — This clam is thinner than the quahog, about $3^1/_2$ inches long, oval in shape and chalky white/gray. The shells are thin and fragile. Soft-shell clams are found on most coasts in the Northern Hemisphere. In the New England area they are found in the sand and gathered at low tide. In the Mid-Atlantic States, they are found farther out to sea and are gathered by dredges. On the West Coast, they are plentiful from Alaska to California. Meat is tender and delicious. Can be eaten raw, broiled in their shells, pan-fried, or in soups, but are at their best steamed.

**COCKLES** (a relative of the oyster)

The original European cockle is not found in the United States. On the East Coast, the *Giant Atlantic Cockle* is found, often measuring better than 5 inches; it is strong-tasting. On the Pacific Coast, the small or nutritious *Basket Cockle* is found from Alaska to California. They average 3 inches in size, with a slightly tough texture but a tasty delicate flavor, and are usually steamed. Both East and West Coast cockles have deep, even ridges that spread out to the scalloped rims of their shells. They are easier to gather than clams because they have no necks, and cannot burrow deeply into the sand.

## MUSSELS

Mussels are almost always cooked, either steamed, fried, or stewed. Mussels can be poisonous if their environment is tainted, yet this rarely has been true of the blue mussel. The *Blue Mussel* is plentiful on the East Coast. The *West Coast Mussel* is a different story; it is dangerous to eat from May to October due to the presence of a plankton, called ganyaulax, in the water. A poison from this plankton, saxitoxin, builds up in the mussel's liver to levels dangerous when ingested by humans. The Mediterranean has a larger and distinct species of mussel, the *Provencal Mussel*, whose flesh is more red than orange, and the *Bearded Mussel*. These are eaten raw. Freshwater mussels are rare.

*Cleaning Mussels and Clams*

Before cooking mussels and clams, you must clean the sand out of their interiors. Sort through mussels and clams, throwing out any that are open or that feel lighter than the rest. Also throw out the ones that are too heavy. Scrub with brush under water, scrape off the beard which protrudes from the closed shell halves of mussels. Put mussels or clams into bucket of water to soak along with ³/₄ cup corn meal and ¹/₄ cup salt to help cleanse sand out. Let soak overnight. If you want to hasten the purging process, add pepper to the water with salt and cornmeal. The clams or mussels will pump faster and an 8-hour job will be done in 3.

*Clams in the Half Shell*

After soaking clams and rinsing, cut shells open, leave clam in half shell, and bread the clam in cornmeal. In a skillet, heat 2 Tablespoons olive oil. Fry clams, clam side down, 3-5 minutes. Oysters and clams are easily opened when washed in cold water, placed in a plastic bag and put in the freezer for about 1 hour.

*Fried Geoduck Steak*

Cut trimmed body of clam into steaks $1/4$ inch thick, pound each steak lightly to tenderize. Sauté in olive oil and garlic for about 20 seconds on each side. Optional: Dip steak into egg and dredge in flour before sautéeing.

## ABALONE

Abalone is a lean, white, very tough muscle meat with a distinctive, delicious flavor. Unless pounded or sliced very thin, it will be tough. Cleaned raw abalone can be kept up to one week if immersed in fresh cold water and refrigerated. Water must be changed daily. Heat toughens abalone, so when cooking, heat only until thoroughly warmed. 1 pound = 3-4 servings.

# PASTA PRIMAVERA WITH SALMON

6 servings

A delicious lowfat entrée.

1½ cups mushrooms — sliced
2 Tablespoons onion — chopped
2 Tablespoons olive oil
1 Tablespoon flour
⅛ teaspoon dried basil
⅛ teaspoon dried oregano
½ cup lowfat milk
¾ pound salmon — cooked and flaked
¾ cup yellow squash — sliced, cooked until crisp and tender
½ cup fresh peas — partially cooked (thawed frozen may be used)
½ cup tomato — diced
1 Tablespoon fresh parsley — minced
1 Tablespoon white wine — optional
8 ounces spinach fettuccine or spaghetti — cooked and drained
Salt — optional
Pepper
Lemon wedges

Sauté mushrooms and onions in oil. Add flour, basil, and oregano;
cook and stir 1 minute. Add milk gradually, cooking and stirring
until sauce thickens. Add salmon, squash, peas, tomato, parsley,
and wine. Heat thoroughly. Toss fettuccine with vegetable mixture.
Season with salt and pepper, place on platter, and garnish with
lemon wedges.

## BROILED SALMON STEAKS

6 servings

*6 salmon steaks*
*2 Tablespoons fresh lemon juice*
*1 teaspoon dried dill*
*1 Tablespoon olive oil*
*Coarsely ground pepper — optional*

Sprinkle each steak with lemon juice. Combine dill and olive oil, rub evenly over steaks, sprinkle each with pepper. Place salmon steaks on a well-greased broiler pan. Broil 4 inches from heat, allowing 10 minutes cooking time per inch of thickness, measured at thickest part, or until salmon flakes with fork. Turn steaks halfway through cooking time.

## BROILED SALMON WITH HERBED LEMON BUTTER

6 servings

*6 salmon steaks*
*¼ cup butter or margarine — melted*
*2 Tablespoons lemon juice*
*2 Tablespoons fresh parsley—chopped*
*¼ teaspoon dried dill weed—crushed*
*¼ teaspoon dried rosemary — crushed*
*⅛ teaspoon coarsely ground pepper*

Line broiler pan with foil or place steaks on a well-greased broiler pan. Combine remaining ingredients, and baste salmon with mixture. Broil 4 inches from heat, allowing 10 minutes cooking time per inch of thickness, measured at thickest part, or until salmon flakes with a fork. Do not turn steaks. Baste several times.

200

# EASY TUNA LUNCH CASSEROLE    4 servings

1 - 6½ ounce can tuna
½ cup fresh mushrooms — sliced, or 4-ounce can, drained
1 can cream of cheddar soup
¼ cup parmesan cheese — grated
¼ cup romano cheese — grated
½ cup 2% milk
2 cups small spiral macaroni
Pepper
Salt — optional

Preheat oven to 350°

In a saucepan, combine tuna, mushrooms, cream of cheddar soup, half of both cheeses, and milk, and stir until heated and combined. Cook macaroni separately until almost done; drain, and place in a baking dish. Pour tuna mixture over macaroni. Sprinkle with remaining cheese. Add pepper and salt. Bake for about 10-12 minutes or until well heated and cheese is melted.

# EASY AND QUICK LUNCH CASSEROLE

3-4 servings

*2 cups pasta — cooked and drained*
*1 cup salmon — use either leftover or canned salmon*
*¼ cup leeks — chopped*
*⅛ cup half-and-half*
*⅓ cup 2% milk*
*½ cup cheese — whatever you have, jarlsberg, romano, parmesan —*
  *grated*
*Pepper*

Preheat oven to 350°

Place cooked pasta in the bottom of a baking dish. In a saucepan, combine salmon, leeks, half-and-half, milk, and ¼ cup of the cheese. Mix well and heat. Pour mixture over pasta. Sprinkle with remaining cheese and bake for 10-15 minutes, or until well heated and cheese on top is melted. Pepper to taste.

Note: Search your refrigerator for leftovers to make up quick and nourishing lunch casseroles that your kids will really like, rather than making a quick dash to the fast food restaurant. The variety of lunch casseroles is endless and all of them can be made ahead of time.


# POACHED SALMON

6 servings

*2 pounds salmon roast*
*2 quarts water*
*½ cup white wine vinegar*
*1 onion — sliced*

*2 or 3 sprigs of fresh parsley*
*1½ teaspoons salt — optional (or use seaweed)*
*1 teaspoon whole peppercorns*
*1 bay leaf*

Wrap salmon in cheesecloth, set aside. Combine remaining ingredients and simmer for 30 minutes. Carefully place cheesecloth-wrapped salmon in poaching liquid. Liquid must cover salmon. Cover pan and simmer, allowing 10 minutes cooking time per inch of thickness, measured at thickest part, or until salmon flakes easily when tested with fork at thickest part. Remove salmon from poaching liquid and discard cheesecloth, remove skin, and serve hot with the following sauce, if desired.

Note: Cheesecloth keeps salmon from falling apart.

---

## *DILL SAUCE*    Approximately ½ cup

*⅓ cup plain nonfat yogurt*
*3 Tablespoons mayonnaise*
*1 Tablespoon parsley — chopped*
*2 teaspoons green onion — diced*
*2 teaspoons fresh lemon juice*
*¼ teaspoon dried dill*
*¼ teaspoon salt — optional*
*Generous dash of Tabasco or hot pepper sauce*

Combine all ingredients and mix thoroughly. Chill at least 1 hour to blend flavors.

# STUFFED SALMON

½ cup onion — chopped
½ cup celery — sliced thin
2 Tablespoons olive oil
2 cups bread crumbs
¼ cup canned smoked oysters — drained and chopped
½ cup canned or fresh clams — drained and chopped
½ cup clam juice
¼ teaspoon dried sage
1 teaspoon dried thyme
Pepper
¼ cup black olives — sliced
1 egg
1½ - 2 pounds whole salmon
1 Tablespoon fresh lemon juice
⅛ teaspoon dried tarragon

Preheat oven to 350°
In a skillet, sauté onion and celery in olive oil for 3 minutes. In a bowl, combine onion mixture, bread crumbs, oysters, clams, clam juice, sage, thyme, pepper, olives, and egg. Mix well. Form 8 Tablespoon-sized balls out of most of the dressing and set aside. Slit salmon down the middle of belly. Do not cut into 2 pieces, only through to skin. Open salmon and sprinkle with fresh lemon juice, pepper, and tarragon. Place salmon in baking dish and place remainder of dressing in center of salmon and close. Place dressing balls around salmon. Cover with foil and seal edges. Bake for approximately 40 minutes (cooking time depends on thickness of fish).

# STEAMED SALMON

4 servings

*¼ teaspoon dried tarragon*
*½ teaspoon dried dill*
*½ teaspoon coarsely ground pepper*
*1½ - 2 pounds salmon steaks or fillets*
*1 Tablespoon fresh lemon juice*

Mix together tarragon, dill, and pepper. Sprinkle on top of salmon. Sprinkle with fresh lemon juice and set aside. In a steamer, bring to boil about 1 inch of water. Place salmon in steamer, lower heat, and cover. Steam 10 minutes per inch of thickness of fish.

# FRITTATA OF SORTS

4 servings

*1 Tablespoon olive oil*
*¼ cup green bell pepper — chopped*
*¼ cup onion — chopped*
*3-4 fresh mushrooms — chopped*
*1 cup cooked salmon — flaked*
*3 cooked prawns — chopped*
*4 eggs (using only 2 yolks to lower cholesterol) — beaten*
*½ cup jarlsberg cheese — sliced or grated*

In a skillet, heat oil. Add green bell pepper, onions, and mushrooms and sauté for 1-2 minutes. Add salmon and prawns, mixing well. Add beaten eggs and scramble mixture until almost done to personal taste. Place cheese on top of mixture, and cover until cheese melts. Serve with toast.

Note: Frittata is attractive when cut into pie-shaped sections.

# *BARBECUED SALMON*

1 pound serves 2

*1 pound salmon — whole or steaks*
*½ teaspoon dried dill*
*2 Tablespoons fresh lemon juice*
*1 Tablespoon butter or margarine*
*½ cup onion — sliced*
*2 Tablespoons oil*
*Pepper*

Wash salmon and pat dry. Cut into steaks if desired. Sprinkle inside of fish (or tops of steaks) with dill, lemon juice, and dot of butter. Arrange overlapping slices of onion in cavity, or on top of steaks. Brush outside of salmon with oil. Sprinkle with pepper. Wrap in foil, sealing edges with double fold. Place on grill over medium-hot coals. Carefully turn foil-wrapped salmon every 5 minutes. Grill 15-20 minutes, depending on thickness of fish. Check for doneness after 15 minutes. To serve, transfer salmon to platter and fold back foil, then cut between bone and meat with spatula. Lift off each serving.

Note: Aluminum foil needed.

A serving of fish is lower in saturated fat than an equal amount of skinless chicken, with about half the cholesterol. Varied, versatile, and quick to prepare, fish merits a place on the menu several times a week.

# SALMON QUICHE WITH SUN-DRIED TOMATOES

4-6 servings

1 partially baked pie shell (see page 270)
¼ cup sun-dried tomatoes — diced
1 Tablespoon olive oil
1 cup fresh mushrooms — sliced
2 Tablespoons onion — chopped
⅓ cup green onion — chopped
1 cup salmon — cooked and flaked (leftover salmon is perfect)
3 Tablespoons parmesan cheese — grated
3 Tablespoons romano cheese — grated
3 eggs — discard 1 yolk
1 cup 2% milk
Pepper

Preheat oven to 450° for pie crust,
then reduce to 350°

Partially bake pie crust. Remove from oven and cover bottom of crust with sun-dried tomatoes. In a skillet, heat oil. Add mushrooms, onions, and green onions, and sauté for 2-3 minutes. Place onion mixture over sun-dried tomatoes. Add flaked salmon, top with grated cheeses. In a blender, combine eggs, milk, and pepper. Blend well. Pour into pie shell. Bake for 40 minutes.

---

## QUICHES

Quiches are practically foolproof, and you can create your own combinations. They can be a first course, a main course, or used as hors d'oeuvres. Quiche ingredients should fill shell no more than three-fourths full to allow room to expand. Crust may be partially baked ahead of time. To test for doneness, use a sharp knife and place in center of quiche. The knife should come out clean. As the quiche cools, it will sink down. Serve hot or cold. It is a great leftover.

# ALMOND SOLE

2-3 servings

1/4 teaspoon sesame seed oil
1 Tablespoon olive oil
2 Tablespoons fresh parsley — chopped
1 Tablespoon garlic — pressed (use pulp)
1 Tablespoon dried dill
Pepper
1/3 cup almonds — slivered
1-1 1/2 pounds sole
2 teaspoons fresh lime juice

In a skillet, heat sesame and olive oils, and sauté parsley for about 1 minute. Add garlic, dill, and pepper, and saute for a couple of minutes. Add almonds. Place sole on top of almonds, sprinkle with lime juice, and cover. Simmer covered for 10 minutes and baste with its own juice for a minute or so. Great served with parsley potatoes and carrot salad.


# FAST AND DELICIOUS
# SALMON TACOS

8 tacos

1 cup cooked salmon — use either leftover or canned salmon
2 Tablespoons black olives — diced
3 Tablespoons onion — diced
3 Tablespoons green taco sauce
8 taco shells
1 cup jarlsberg cheese — grated

Preheat oven to 350°

In a bowl, combine salmon, olives, onion, and green taco sauce. Fill each taco shell with salmon mixture, and top with grated cheese. Place on cookie sheet and bake until cheese melts. Garnish suggestions: Diced tomatoes, avocado slices, or favorite salsa.

## UNCLE BILL'S STEELHEAD ON THE GRILL
3-4 servings

*2 - 4 pound steelhead*
*2 Tablespoons margarine — melted*
*1/4 teaspoon liquid smoke*
*1/2 - 1 teaspoon lemon pepper — depending on taste*

Fillet steelhead, but do not remove the skin, and cut to desired size. In a saucepan, melt margarine. Add liquid smoke, and mix. Brush this butter mixture onto fish, sprinkle with lemon pepper, and let refrigerate for about 1/2 hour. Place on grill (medium-hot coals), meat side down, sear it, turn to skin side down and continue to cook until done (about 10 minutes per inch of thickness).

## UNCLE BILL'S BARBECUED SALMON OR TROUT

*Fish*
*Foil*
*Light margarine*
*Favorite barbecue sauce*

Place fish onto foil, dab with margarine, and brush with favorite sauce. Close foil up tightly and place on grill (medium-hot coals). Allow approximately 10 minutes per inch of thickness.

## SAUTÉED BLACK COD                    2-3 servings

*½ cup onion — sliced*
*1 teaspoon dried thyme*
*1 Tablespoon olive oil*
*1 pound black cod*
*2 Tablespoons fresh lemon juice*
*Pepper*
*1 tomato — sliced*

In a skillet, sauté onions and thyme in olive oil. Add black cod, sprinkling fish with lemon juice and pepper. Lay tomato slices on top of fish, cover, and simmer until fish is done, about 5-10 minutes, depending on thickness of fish.

**210**

# BAKED COD

3-4 servings

*½ cup onion — sliced*
*½ cup celery — sliced*
*2 garlic cloves — pressed*
*1 tomato — sliced*
*1½-2 pounds cod*
*Pepper*
*½ teaspoon dried thyme*
*¼ teaspoon dried basil*
*¼ cup tomato sauce*

Preheat oven to 350°
In a baking dish, place a layer of onion, celery, garlic, and tomato slices. Place cod on top of layer, and cover fish with a repeat layer. Sprinkle with pepper, thyme, and basil. Pour tomato sauce over top of fish. Cover with foil, bake for 20 minutes, remove foil, return to oven 5-10 minutes longer. This recipe is also quite good using Pacific sea bass.

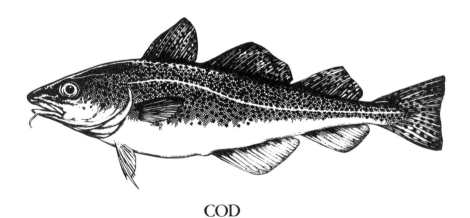

COD

# STUFFED TROUT

2-3 servings

*2 Tablespoons margarine*
*½ cup onion — chopped*
*1 Tablespoon fresh parsley — chopped*
*1 teaspoon fresh thyme — chopped*
*½ cup fresh mushrooms — sliced*
*1 cup fresh shrimp*
*2 whole trout, about 2 pounds total — remove bones*
*2 teaspoons fresh lemon juice*
*1 Tablespoon margarine — melted*

Preheat oven to 400°

In a skillet, melt margarine. Add onions, parsley, thyme, and mushrooms. Sauté until onions are tender. Add shrimp and lemon juice and cook until heated through. Remove from heat. Remove heads from trout, cut down center (not all the way through skin), place ½ of shrimp mixture into center of each trout, close and secure with toothpick. Place into a baking dish, sprinkle fish with fresh lemon juice, drizzle with 1 Tablespoon melted margarine, cover with foil, and bake for 20 minutes. Check for doneness. Two slices of orange and a sprig of parsley make an easy and attractive garnish.

---

### SARDINES

Open a can of sardines and carefully remove fish, transfer to small skillet, add liquid from sardine can and squeeze of fresh lemon juice. Heat thoroughly. Arrange sardines on small toast crackers or bread cut into small sizes. Garnish with lemon.

# HALIBUT PATTIES

6-8 patties

*1½ cups halibut — cooked and flaked (remove bones)*
*¼ cup onion — chopped*
*1 Tablespoon fresh lemon juice*
*½ cup carrots — grated*
*Pepper*
*½ cup cornmeal*
*⅓ cup 2% milk*
*1 egg*
*1½ Tablespoons oil (monounsaturated or polyunsaturated)*

In a bowl, mix all ingredients and form patties. In a skillet, heat oil, brown patties on both sides and serve warm.

# HALIBUT CURRY SALAD

4 small servings

*½ pound halibut — cooked*
*1 cup whole kernel corn — cooked and removed from cob*
*¼ cup dill pickles — chopped*
*3 Tablespoons mayonnaise — without sugar and preservatives*
*½ cup onions — chopped*
*Pepper*
*½-1 teaspoon curry (if not familiar with curry, be cautious — add*
*    just a little at first)*

Mix all ingredients together and chill. Serve on lettuce or raw spinach, sprinkled with cheese, or serve with crackers. Also great on a variety salad plate.

# HALIBUT SAUTÉ

4 servings

*1 pound halibut, thawed if frozen*
*1½ Tablespoons olive oil*
*1 cup EACH carrots, celery, green onions, and broccoli florets —*
*    sliced thin*
*¼ teaspoon fresh ginger root — grated (¼ teaspoon ground ginger*
*    may be substituted)*
*¼ cup chicken stock (or water)*
*2 teaspoons cornstarch*
*1 teaspoon lemon or lime peel — grated*
*Pepper*
*Low-sodium soy sauce*
*Red bell pepper strips and sesame seeds for garnish*

Remove bones from halibut. Cut into 1-inch pieces. In a skillet, heat oil. Add halibut cubes and cook until almost done. Remove halibut from skillet and set aside. Add vegetables to skillet and cook until crisp-tender. Return halibut to skillet, together with ginger, stock, cornstarch, and lemon or lime peel. Mix well and simmer until sauce is thickened and halibut flakes easily when tested with a fork. Season to taste with pepper and low-sodium soy sauce. Add red bell pepper strips and sesame seeds for garnish.

# ALASKA WHITEFISH STEW

6-8 servings

*1½ pounds cod, pollock, or rockfish fillets*
*1 Tablespoon olive oil*
*1½ cups green bell peppers — chopped*
*1 cup carrots — sliced thin*
*¾ cup onion — chopped*

*1 large garlic clove — minced*
*1 - 28 ounce can tomatoes*
*1 - 12 ounce can tomato juice*
*1½ teaspoons Worcestershire sauce*
*1 teaspoon dried basil*
*½ teaspoon brown sugar*
*½ cup white wine or fish stock*

Cut fish into 1-inch pieces. Heat oil in large pot. Add green bell peppers, carrots, onion, and garlic, and sauté until onion is tender. Add tomatoes, tomato juice, Worcestershire sauce, basil, and sugar. Bring to a boil; simmer, covered, 10 minutes. Add wine and fish. Simmer 8 minutes longer on medium heat, or until fish flakes easily when tested with a fork.

# BARBECUED TROUT

*Foil wrap*
*Dab of margarine*
*Trout — cleaned*
*Few onion slices*
*Tomato slice*
*Fresh lemon juice*
*Pepper*

Place margarine and trout in foil; lay onion and tomato slices on top, sprinkle with lemon juice and pepper. Wrap tightly and place on grill (medium-hot coals) until done. Allow about 10 minutes per inch of thickness, measured at thickest part.

# BAKED SEA PERCH

2-3 servings

*1 pound sea perch*
*½ cup white wine*
*⅓ cup onion — sliced thin*
*Coarsely ground pepper*
*3 garlic cloves — minced and chopped fine*
*Pinch of dried tarragon*
*¼ teaspoon dried thyme*
*2 Tablespoons green onion — chopped*
*1 tomato — sliced thick*

Preheat oven to 350°

Place all ingredients into a bowl and refrigerate 30 minutes to 1 hour. Place fish and marinade into baking dish and bake 20-25 minutes or until fish is done.

---

## HERBS AND SPICES

Herbs and spices can be combined in creative ways to make seafood recipes more flavorful. Instead of using the salt shaker, try cooking with herbs and spices to enhance the flavor. If unfamiliar with herbs and spices, start by combining ¼ teaspoon of 1 or 2 herbs or spices per pound of seafood.

| | | |
|---|---|---|
| Allspice | Dill seed | Oregano |
| Basil | Dill weed | Paprika |
| Bay leaf | Fennel seed | Parsley |
| Cayenne pepper | Garlic powder | Rosemary |
| Celery seed | Marjoram | Saffron |
| Chervil | Mustard | Tarragon |
| Curry powder | Nutmeg | Thyme |

Other seasonings to use with seafood are garlic, lemon juice, and wine.

# FRESH PERCH FOR TWO

2 servings

*½ cup white wine*
*½ cup onion — sliced thin*
*3 small cloves garlic — pressed or minced*
*⅛ teaspoon dried tarragon*
*¼ teaspoon dried thyme*
*¼ cup green onion — chopped*
*1 tomato — sliced thick*
*1 pound perch*

Preheat oven to 350°

In a bowl, combine white wine, onion, garlic, tarragon, thyme, green onion, and tomato. Add fish and marinate in refrigerator for 1 hour. Remove fish and place in a baking dish. Pour marinade over fish and arrange vegetables on top of fish. Cover with foil, bake for 30 minutes. Cooking time depends on thickness of fillets.

## SNAPPER WITH MUSHROOMS AND ASPARAGUS

2-3 servings

*¼ cup onion — sliced*
*½ cup green pepper — sliced*
*¾ cup fresh mushrooms — sliced*
*Pepper — optional*
*1 pound snapper*
*1 dozen asparagus spears — washed*
*1 teaspoon lemon juice*
*⅛ teaspoon dried tarragon*

Preheat oven to 350°

In the bottom of a baking dish, place onions, green peppers, and mushrooms. Sprinkle with pepper. Lay fish on top of vegetables. Place a layer of asparagus spears over fish, sprinkle with lemon juice and tarragon. Cover with foil and seal edges. Bake for 20-25 minutes.

## SNAPPER WITH ASPARAGUS AND PARMESAN CHEESE

2-3 servings

*1 Tablespoon olive oil*
*½ cup onion — sliced*
*1 garlic clove — chopped*
*1 tomato — sliced*
*1-1½ pounds snapper*
*1 Tablespoon lemon juice*
*Pepper*
*1 dozen asparagus spears — washed*
*3 Tablespoons parmesan cheese — freshly grated*

**218**

Preheat oven to 350°

In the bottom of a baking dish, place olive oil, onion, and garlic. Cover with sliced tomato. Lay fish on top of tomato slices and sprinkle with half the lemon juice and pepper. Place a layer of asparagus over fish. Sprinkle with remaining lemon juice, pepper, and cheese. Cover with foil and seal edges. Bake for 25-30 minutes.

---

# UNCLE RAY'S POTATO FISHCAKES

2-3 servings

*1 cup well-cooked fish fillets — ¹/₂ cup white (halibut, ling cod, rockfish) and ¹/₂ cup salmon*
*1 cup mashed potatoes*
*1 egg — beaten*
*¹/₄ cup green onion — chopped*
*Salt and pepper to taste*
*Dash of soy sauce*
*¹/₄ teaspoon nutmeg*
*1 cup polyunsaturated oil*

Finely flake fish. Combine all ingredients except oil. Heat oil in a skillet to approximately 350° and drop mixture by spoonfuls into oil. Dip spoon in oil between scoops so mixture slides easily off spoon. Fry until golden brown on both sides. Serve with tartar sauce. This is a tasty way to clean out the freezer. Aunt Diane's variation: Mix grated cheese into the mixture.

## RAY'S TERIYAKI FISH FRY

2 servings

*⅓ cup low-sodium soy sauce*
*2 heaping Tablespoons brown sugar*
*1 teaspoon ground ginger*
*1 teaspoon dry mustard*
*¼ cup dry red wine*
*1 garlic clove — crushed*
*1 pound fish fillets — halibut, salmon or rockfish*
*1 cup polyunsaturated oil*
*Sesame seeds*

Combine all ingredients except sesame seeds and oil. Marinate fish in the mixture for about 2 hours in refrigerator. In a skillet, heat oil. Add fillets. Sprinkle with sesame seeds. Cover and cook 3-5 minutes. Turn fillets, sprinkle with more sesame seeds, and cook about 5 more minutes. (Allow 10 minutes cooking time per inch of thickness.)

## SIMPLE BLACK COD

2-3 servings

*1 Tablespoon olive oil*
*½ cup onion — sliced*
*1 teaspoon dried thyme*
*1½-2 pounds black cod*
*Pepper*
*1 teaspoon fresh lemon juice*
*1 tomato — sliced*

In a skillet, heat oil. Add onions and thyme and sauté for a minute or so. Add fish, sprinkle with pepper and lemon juice, and lay slices of tomato over fish. Cover, cook 4-5 minutes, remove cover, turn fish over and cook 4-5 minutes longer.

---

# SNAPPER WITH MUSHROOMS 2 servings

*1 Tablespoon olive oil*
*3 garlic cloves — peeled and diced*
*2 Tablespoons parsley — chopped*
*3 Tablespoons fresh lemon juice*
*1 pound snapper — rinse and pat dry*
*Pepper*
*1 cup fresh mushrooms — sliced*

In a skillet, heat oil. Add garlic, parsley, and ½ of lemon juice, and sauté 2-3 minutes. Place snapper in skillet and sprinkle with remainder of lemon juice and pepper. Add mushrooms and cook 10-15 minutes, depending on thickness of snapper.

# RONDA'S FAST BAKED HALIBUT
## (OR SNAPPER)

Not lowfat, but delicious.

Preheat oven to 375°

Marinate fish in white wine about 1-1$^{1}/_{2}$ hours.
Dredge in cracker crumbs and place in an oiled baking dish. Mix half sour cream and half mayonnaise, pour over top of fish, and sprinkle with remaining crumbs left over from dredging. Bake for 20 minutes.

Note: May substitute cheese instead of cracker crumbs.

# ROUGHY WITH LIME JUICE          2-3 servings

*1 Tablespoon olive oil*
*2 Tablespoons fresh dill — minced*
*4 garlic cloves — pressed (discard pulp)*
*3 Tablespoons fresh lime juice*
*$^{1}/_{4}$ cup peanuts — unsalted*
*1-1$^{1}/_{2}$ pounds roughy*
*Pepper*

In a skillet, heat olive oil. Add dill, garlic, half of lime juice, and peanuts. Sauté 2-3 minutes. Sprinkle remaining lime juice over fish, then sprinkle with pepper. Add fish to skillet, cover, and cook fish 3-5 minutes, remove cover and continue cooking until fish is done (about 3-5 minutes longer).

**222**

# SEAFOOD BANQUET

4-5 servings

*2 Dungeness crabs — cooked (see page 193)*
*2 pounds fresh prawns with shells — cooked (see note, page 225)*
*2 lobsters — cooked*
*Clams (optional) — steamed*

Cook crabs, prawns, and lobsters. Clean crab, break up lobster. Place all seafood into a LARGE serving bowl and serve with individual servings of melted butter and cocktail sauce or a favorite sauce of your own. Also delicious with a platter of cooked fresh corn on the cob and a fruit salad, when in season.

# SAUTÉED PRAWNS

4 servings

*1 Tablespoon unsalted butter*
*2 garlic cloves — pressed*
*4 green onions — chopped*
*1 cup fresh mushrooms — sliced thick*
*1 pound fresh prawns — after shelling*
*⅓ cup white wine*

In a skillet, combine butter, garlic, onions, and mushrooms. Sauté 2-3 minutes. Add shelled prawns and white wine. Simmer 5-8 minutes on medium-low heat, just until they are opaque. Can be served over rice or with pasta.

# SHRIMP QUICHE

1 pie crust — partially baked (see page 270)
3/4 cup jarlsberg cheese — shredded
2 teaspoons olive oil
1/2 cup onions — sliced
3/4 cup fresh mushrooms — sliced
1 cup fresh or frozen shrimp
3 eggs — discard 1 or 2 yolks
1 teaspoon Dijon mustard
1/2 cup whipping cream
1/2 cup 2% or nonfat milk
Pepper

Preheat oven to 450° for pie crust, then reduce to 350°

Partially bake pie crust. Remove from oven and cover bottom of crust with jarslberg cheese. In a skillet, heat olive oil and sauté onions and mushrooms for 2 minutes. Add shrimp and stir. Drain and arrange over cheese in crust. In blender, beat eggs. Add mustard, cream, milk, and pepper and blend well. Pour into crust over shrimp mixture. Bake for 35-40 minutes. Quiche is done when knife inserted 1 inch from edge comes out clean. Remove from oven and let stand 10 minutes before cutting. Cut into wedges.

# PRAWNS

*Prawns*
*2 Tablespoons olive oil*
*Fresh parsley — chopped*
*Pinch of cayenne pepper*

Clean prawns and peel to tails (leave tails on). In a skillet, heat oil. Add prawns, sprinkle with parsley and a pinch of cayenne. Sauté until prawns are done, no longer than 5 minutes. (It cannot be over-emphasized that shrimp should be cooked only long enough to give them firmness and color, 3-5 minutes, just until they are opaque.)

Note: When boiling prawns, try adding 3 Tablespoons pickling spice (remove the cinnamon) to the boiling water before adding prawns, or use milk instead of water for a sweeter flavor.
Steam cleaned clams in milk instead of water — it makes its own clam chowder.

# SNOW CRAB PAELLA

6 servings

*1 pound Snow crab clusters, single cut legs or split legs — thaw if
    necessary*
*1 Tablespoon olive oil*
*1 pound chicken thighs — remove skin*
*1 large onion — chopped*
*6 ounces nitrate-free Italian sausage — sliced*
*1½ cups uncooked long grain rice*
*4 cups chicken broth*
*1 teaspoon salt — optional*
*½ teaspoon paprika*
*1 package (10 ounces) frozen peas — thawed and drained*

Rinse crab under cool water and cut into serving-sized pieces. Score
backs of leg sections, using large, heavy knife or slit with kitchen
shears. Heat oil in large skillet. Add chicken and cook 20 minutes,
turning to brown all sides. Remove from skillet. Sauté onion and
sausage about 5 minutes. Add rice and sauté until lightly browned.
Return chicken to skillet. Add broth and seasonings. Simmer covered for 30 minutes. Add crab and peas; cover and cook about 5
minutes longer or until thoroughly heated.

# SNOW CRAB FRITTATA

6 servings

*1 Tablespoon olive oil*
*1 garlic clove — pressed*
*²/₃ onion — chopped*
*1 cup zucchini — chopped*
*¹/₂ cup mushrooms — sliced*
*3 eggs*
*¹/₂ cup nonfat milk*
*¹/₄ cup parmesan cheese — grated*
*¹/₄ teaspoon pepper*
*6-8 ounces snow crab meat — thaw if necessary, drain and slice*
*Garnish — tomato rose and Snow crab claw*

Preheat oven to 350°

Heat oil in a large skillet. Add garlic, onion, zucchini, and mushrooms. Sauté until tender, about 5 minutes. Beat together eggs, milk, cheese, and pepper. In an oiled 1¹/₂-quart casserole (or ovenproof skillet), alternate layers of crab and zucchini mixture, and pour egg mixture over all. Bake for 20-25 minutes or until firm.

Note: This is a great recipe for a brunch. Loaded with nutritious vegetables and seafood, this egg dish feeds six people with just three eggs. If you're trying to cut back on eggs, this recipe fits the bill, with only half an egg per serving.

# CRAB WITH RED SAUCE

Approximately 1¹/₄ cups sauce

*1¹/₂ lbs. crab clusters, single cut legs or split — cooked*
*2 Tablespoons onion — minced*
*1 garlic clove — minced*
*1 Tablespoon margarine*
*1 - 8 ounce can tomato sauce*
*¹/₄ cup ketchup*
*¹/₄ teaspoon dried oregano — crushed*

Rinse crab in cool water and cut into serving-sized pieces. Score backs of leg sections with heavy knife or shears. Sauté onion and garlic in margarine until tender. Stir in remaining ingredients except crab. Simmer 5 minutes. Serve hot with chilled or hot crab.

---

### SEAWEED

Seaweeds come in many shapes, colors, and sizes. Most seaweeds are inedible, but some are very good, such as Agar-Agar, Nori, Oulse, Irish Moss, Sea Lettuce, Hijike, Kelp, Laver, Spirulina, Kombu, Algin, and Wakame. Seaweed can be used as a vegetable, or in soups, sushi, stir-fry, seafood appetizers, even sprinkled on pizza before baking. The Japanese have been using seaweeds for over 300 years and have over 20 kinds of cuisine in which it is used.

The real benefit of seaweed is its outstanding mineral content. Iron, calcium, phosphorus, potassium, and iodine, essential nutrients our bodies need, are widely abundant in seaweeds. Most types provide a good supply of protein, vitamins A and B, with small quantities of vitamin C and are low in fat. Seaweed is a GREAT salt substitute!

Be sure to wash seaweed before using to remove extra salt and sand or tiny shells which may cling to fronds.

# COLD LOBSTER/CRAB PASTA

3-4 servings

*1 medium-sized lobster — cooked, cleaned, and separated*
*1 Dungeness crab — cooked, cleaned, and separated (see pages 192-193)*
*8-10 ounces of red bell pepper pasta (see page 284) or use your favorite pasta*
*1½ Tablespoons olive oil*
*2-3 garlic cloves — chopped and pressed (using pulp)*
*⅓ cup leeks — chopped*
*½ cup pine nuts*
*2 Tablespoons fresh lemon juice*

Precook lobster and crab. Cook pasta. In a skillet, heat olive oil and margarine. Add garlic, leeks, and pine nuts. Sauté 2-3 minutes. Add chopped cooked lobster, crab, and fresh lemon juice. Mix well and cook about 1 minute. Remove from heat. Toss with pasta. Chill and serve. Also very good served warm.

**229**

# SQUID

This exotic member of the shellfish family has no outer shell and swims freely in the ocean, its long tentacles trailing behind it. There are about 350 different species of squid, ranging from tiny creatures a few inches long to giant squids which reach over 60 feet in length. More than 80% of the squid is edible. There are dozens of ways to serve squid, sautéed as in the recipe below, grilled and sprinkled with fresh lemon juice, stuffed, or cut into rings and fried, to name just a few of the ways. Squid is available fresh, frozen, dried, or canned. Do not be squeamish about cleaning squid: Just think of the marvelous flavor, and the price per pound saved cleaning your own. You will do just fine.

*To Clean Squid:*
1. Hold under cold running water, rub and pull off the purplish membrane to expose the white meat.
2. Pull body from mantle (outer sac), then pull the long clear quill (technically its shell) and contents from inside the mantle and discard. Rinse mantle with water and drain briefly.
3. Cut body between eyes and tentacles (discard eyes and material attached).
4. Pop out and discard the round, hard beak in the center of the tentacles.

Note: Leave the purplish skin on the tentacles — it adds color to your dish.

# SAUTÉED SQUID WITH MUSHROOMS AND PEPPERS

2-3 servings

1 Tablespoon olive oil
4 large garlic cloves — peeled and sliced
1/2 cup onions — sliced
2 Tablespoons fresh parsley — chopped
1 Tablespoon fresh lemon juice
1-1 1/2 pounds squid — cleaned and sliced into rings
1 cup fresh mushrooms — sliced
1/3 cup yellow bell pepper — quartered and sliced thin
1/3 cup red bell pepper — quartered and sliced thin
1 - 8 ounce can salt-free tomato sauce
1/2 cup water
2 teaspoons flour
1/4-1/2 teaspoon dried thyme — depending on taste

In a skillet, heat oil, combine garlic, onions, and parsley. Sauté about 2 minutes. Add lemon juice, squid, mushrooms, bell peppers, and tomato sauce, and simmer over medium-low heat. In a small bowl, mix 1/2 cup water and 2 teaspoons flour together. Add to squid mixture, stir in thyme, and simmer, covered, on medium-low heat 8-10 minutes longer. Great served with rice or pasta.

# GEODUCK STEW

2 teaspoons olive oil
2 garlic cloves — pressed, diced
½ cup onion — chopped
⅓ cup celery — chopped
⅓ cup green bell pepper — chopped
½ cup carrots — diced
4 strips nitrite-free bacon — diced, cooked
1 cup clam juice
1 cup fish stock
2 cups tomato sauce
1 cup chili sauce
2 Tablespoons fresh lemon juice
1 teaspoon filé powder
½ teaspoon dried thyme
½ pound geoduck clams (or other clams) — diced
½ pound salmon (or cod) — cut into small chunks
1 - 10 ounce package frozen okra — slightly thawed

In a large saucepan over medium-high heat, combine oil, garlic, onion, celery, green bell pepper, and carrots and sauté until onions are soft. Stir in bacon, clam juice, fish stock, tomato sauce, chili sauce, lemon juice, filé powder, and thyme. Simmer over low heat for 5 minutes. Add clams, salmon, and okra. Continue to cook over low heat, covered, until okra is tender and stew is heated through, about 15-20 minutes.

# CLAM LINGUINI

4-6 servings

In the time it takes to cook the pasta, you can prepare this delicious sauce.

*1 Tablespoon unsalted butter or margarine*
*4 garlic cloves — minced*
*2 Tablespoons leeks — chopped*
*1 cup clam juice — drained from clams*
*3 Tablespoons unbleached white flour*
*¾ cup nonfat milk*
*¼ cup half-and-half*
*4 Tablespoons parmesan cheese — grated*
*½ pound jumbo shrimp — rinsed and drained*
*3 - 6 ounce cans clams — chopped*
*2 - 8 ounce packages of linguini — cooked*
*Fresh parsley for garnish*

In a skillet, melt butter. Add garlic and leeks and sauté a minute or so. Add clam juice and simmer on low heat. Meanwhile, combine flour and nonfat milk and mix well. Add flour-milk mixture, half-and-half, and parmesan cheese to sauté. Let simmer on low heat until sauce thickens, stirring often. When sauce reaches desired thickness add shrimp and clams. Continue to let simmer until shrimp and clams are well heated. Place drained cooked pasta into a large serving dish, place ⅔ of the sauce over pasta, sprinkle with a little fresh parsley, and serve. Use last third of the sauce to freshen up pasta for seconds.

# NOTES

# NOTES

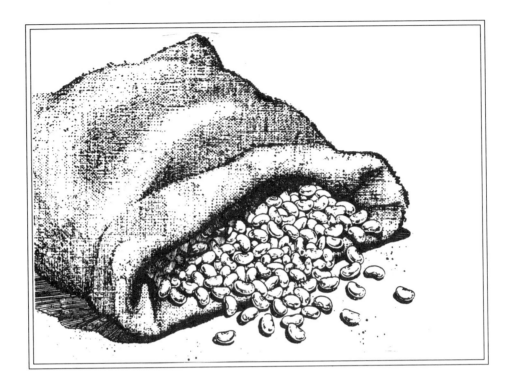

# GRAINS/BEANS

# TAKE A FITNESS BREAK

Break up the work day; before lunching take an exercise break. Walk or jog for 15-20 minutes. Challenge a friend to a game of racquetball or handball. Eat a light lunch — salads or seafood are good choices — while avoiding sautées in margarine or oil, and frying with batter coatings. Isn't it nice to know that reducing cancer may be one of exercise's healthy virtues? So keep your legs pumping, waist bending and twisting, arms swinging. Whatever you choose to do KEEP ACTIVE!! You will gain better health. Your heart will work less even at rest. By beating more slowly, it pumps more with each stroke.

Children need exercise too. Sixty percent of America's youth are overweight and in poor cardiovascular shape, according to the President's Council on Physical Fitness. Children need exercises that produce balanced increases in muscle strength and endurance. The best exercise for children is vigorous play. Help them by taking them to the park, monitoring their T.V. hours, and being involved.

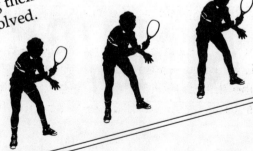

# GRAINS

Grains have been staple foods in almost all cultures for thousands of years. They are a common source of carbohydrates, and the cheapest source of protein, calories, and nutrients. Among the main cultivated grains are rice, wheat, rye, millet, corn, oats, and buckwheat. A grain is made up of 3 basic parts: The bran (or hull), the outer layers of the kernel that protect the grain; the germ ("heart" of the seed) that provides the nutrients; and the endosperm, the center of the grain or the starchy bulk.

A grain is "whole" when it comes with all 3 parts intact. The grain is "refined" to varying degrees by removing the bran (hulling) or removing the germ (degerminating). The more the grain is refined, the more bran and germ are removed, and the lower the nutritional value becomes.

Many of the products available to us today are extremely refined, with most or all of the bran and germ removed — for example, white bread, white flour, white rice, and degerminated cornmeal. Whole grains are very important to our diets and good health. I have listed the main grains and their nutritional value, along with some new recipes to help you start adding them to your daily diet. Once you taste the delicious flavor, texture, and crunch of whole grains, and think about all their nutritional benefits, you will find them hard to resist.

For added information on the benefits of fiber in your diet, see page 33-36.

Note: When buying a commercial whole-grain bread, read the label carefully to make sure you are getting whole grain. A whole-grain bread should list 100% whole wheat flour, or possibly cracked wheat, as its first ingredient (ingredients are listed in order of weight).

# AMARANTH

The ancient Aztecs were nourished on this high-energy grain which is a complete protein, provides a high level of the essential amino acid lysine, and is high in calcium, with traces of a variety of other vitamins and minerals. Amaranth has a pleasant nutty flavor. The grain can be parched and ground coarsely for use as a cereal, or ground finely into flour, or powdered and used in nourishing drinks. To boost the protein of recipes that call for flour, add $1/4$ cup amaranth flour. Amaranth is now finding its way into the grocery stores. If you cannot find it, check the health food stores.

# BARLEY

Preliminary studies indicate that barley helps lower blood cholesterol. Studies have shown that oats and oat bran also help lower blood cholesterol, but barley appears to have more of the cholesterol-suppressing substance. Barley provides phosphorus, potassium, iron, and calcium. However, it has a marginal protein content, with a low level of lysine. Barley can absorb large amounts of water without losing its shape, and is wonderfully satisfying in stews, soups, and vegetable dishes.

**Cracked Barley** (grits or groats) — Makes a delicious blend with other grits in cereal. *To cook:* 2 parts water/1 part grits. Bring water to a boil, add grits, return to a boil, lower heat, and cook, covered, about 20-25 minutes. To cut cooking time, soak grits overnight.

**Pearled Barley** — Is processed to remove the hull and bran, and some of the germ.

**Barley Flour** — Gluten-free. Makes a great wheat substitute for those who are allergic to wheat. Has a bland flavor, but toasting it before adding to bread dough will enhance the flavor.

# BULGUR

Wheat grains that have been parboiled, dried, partially de-branned, and then either finely or coarsely ground. The U.S. Department of Agriculture has developed a process that retains almost all

240

of the niacin, minerals, and the nutritious aleurone layers of the original wheat grain. Bulgur is nutritious, versatile, quick to prepare, and has a nutty flavor. It is great as a meat extender, added to fish patties, as a rice substitute, in soups, salads, and baked goods.

*To cook:* 2 parts water/1 part bulgur, cook, covered, 10 minutes, or soak in water overnight to shorten cooking time.

## *BUCKWHEAT*

Buckwheat is not a true grain, but belongs to the polygonaceae family, related to rhubarb. Buckwheat is an extremely nutritious cereal with complete protein, high in lysine and low in methionine. It is rich in vitamins and minerals, especially magnesium, manganese, and potassium, and low in sodium. Buckwheat is wheat-free, but read the labels on buckwheat products to make sure wheat has not been added. Buckwheat is quick cooking, light or dark brown in color, and has a nutty flavor.

**Whole Buckwheat Grain** (berries) — These are steamed, dried, and milled to remove hulls. The Japanese call their product Soba Mai. Can be cooked like rice in cereals, or added to breads.

**Buckwheat Seeds** (groats or kasha) — Grain is stone ground just enough to crack the hull without actually grinding the seeds. Use in cereals and soups.

---

### GLUTEN

A nutritious protein containing gliadin, found in hard grains, which gives dough its elastic quality.

*A high gluten content* usually results in a flour with a high rising, high water-absorbing quality; it can make a large volume of dough with a light, open texture, such as is needed in bread.

*A low gluten content*, soft starchy flour, usually makes the best cakes.

When you are making yeast-raised bread with a mixture of gluten and non-gluten (or low gluten) flours (such as rye, buckwheat, millet, cornmeal, triticale, or rice flour), always mix in the gluten flour first. This enables the gluten do its work more easily, and helps shorten kneading time.

---

**Buckwheat Grits** — Coarsely ground groats, which have a shorter cooking time than the whole grain.

**Buckwheat Flour** — Gluten-free. Great in pancakes, noodles, breads, and waffles. Because buckwheat flour is gluten-free and rather heavy in breads, it is sometimes mixed with wheat flour.

*To cook:*

Grits — 2 parts water/1 part grits. Bring water to a boil, add grits, return to a boil, lower heat, cook covered 10-15 minutes.

Groats — 2 parts water/1 part groats. Bring water to a boil, add groats, return to a boil, lower heat, cook covered 20-30 minutes. Overnight soaking will shorten cooking time.

## CORN *(Maize)*

Corn is the only grain that contains vitamin A. It also provides notable amounts of B-complex vitamins, calcium, magnesium, phosphorus, iron, potassium, and zinc. Corn is rich in carbohydrates and higher in fat than rice or wheat, but lacking in quantity or quality of protein. Even though corn is normally 10% protein, half this protein is poorly utilized by the body. Corn is also low in lysine and tryptophane, essential amino acids the body cannot manufacture. Corn has a sweet flavor.

**Corn Husks** — Sold ready-prepared for use in making tamales.

**Corn Grains** (whole corn on or off the cob) — Whole grain corn is great alone or in salads, casseroles, soups, fritters, or dried for popping.

**Hominy** — Hulled kernels of soaked, dried corn. Use as a vegetable or cereal.

**Grits** (groats) — Hominy ground into large pieces. Use in cereals and breads.

**Corn Flakes** — Rolled and toasted hominy. Use in cereals.

**Cornmeal** — Degerminated corn, coarsely ground. Use in breads, muffins, tamales, pancakes, even pizza crust. Must be enriched with B vitamins because germ is removed.

**Stone-Ground Cornmeal** — Corn slowly ground between buhr stones, rather than high speed rollers. The entire corn germ remains in the meal. Used for cereals and breads.

**Corn Germ** — Valuable source of B vitamins, high in iron, with a tasty flavor and crunchy texture. Can be used in a variety of recipes, cereals, stuffings, breads, or cookies.

**Corn Flour** — Finely ground corn, frequently used in flat breads, tortillas, and cookies.

**Cornstarch** — A fine, granular or powdery starch made from corn and used in cooking and to make corn sugar, corn syrup, etc.

## MILLET

Millet is one of the most nutritious foods known to man. It is a complete protein, containing all the essential amino acids, and is richer in vitamins and minerals than any other grain except wild rice. Millet is gluten-free, and very alkaline, an unusual characteristic among grains, and very important for those on special diets. Even people with rice allergies can usually eat millet. Millet contains all the essential vitamins and minerals, especially vitamin B complex, calcium, potassium, iron, and magnesium, plus all the important trace elements. Millet varies in size, shape, and color. One cup of millet provides 34 grams of the highest grade protein (about one day's adult requirement). The millet plant is unusual because it can survive without water for long periods of time by rolling up its leaves around the seed and stalk, preventing water loss. When it rains, the growing process resumes.

**Millet Grain** (berries) — Use only hulled millet; the hull is very hard and useless for human consumption. Hulled millet retains all its protein, vitamins, and minerals. It is a popular rice substitute, and adds crunchy richness to breads, soups, or desserts. *To cook:* 2 parts water/1 part millet. Cook, covered, 20-30 minutes, or to cut cooking time in half, soak millet overnight.

**Millet Grits** (groats) — Coarsely ground millet. Use in cereals and breads.

**Millet Flour** — Gluten-free. Slightly heavy flour, with a somewhat bitter flavor. Best when mixed with other flours.

## OATS

Traditionally, wheat has been more popular than oats as a source of the dietary fiber believed to be beneficial in the prevention of cancer and other diseases. However, recent research is lending credence to the beneficial effects of oats on health and well being. Oat bran is actually the part of the crushed oat grain left after milling, and is not merely bran, but 3-4 layers of cells called aleurone layers. Much of the vitamins, minerals, and protein of oat bran is concentrated in these cell layers. Oat bran is high in thiamine, iron, phosphorus, and protein. According to the American Institute for Cancer Research (AICR), oat bran is water-soluble, unlike wheat bran, because it has high concentrations of water-soluble gums. Oat bran's water solubility may give it broader health effects than wheat bran. Wheat bran mostly affects the gastrointestinal tract, acting as a laxative and helping to prevent colorectal cancer. Oat bran, on the other hand, has been shown to lower blood cholesterol, normalize blood sugar levels in diabetics, and may even help reduce blood pressure. Uncooked oats may be more beneficial for lowering blood sugar and blood pressure. Oats, however, should not replace other sources of dietary fiber such as fresh vegetables, fresh fruits, and unrefined grains and beans.

Oats or oat bran can easily be added to your diet, aside from eating them cooked or raw as cereals. You can add oat bran to your morning juice, use it as a thickener in stews and soups, or as a breading for fish and chicken; whole oats can be added to baked goods, meat loaf, granolas, pancakes, and even pizza crust. Oats provide a chewy, moist texture and a sweet flavor.

**Oat Groats** — Whole grain oats with only the hull removed. They have a relatively high protein level compared to other grains.

**Steel Cut Oats** (sometimes called "Irish" or "Scotch" oats) — Are whole grains that have been broken into several pieces for quicker cooking as a delicious hot cereal with a nutty texture.

**Oat Flakes** — Are extra large, heavy, white whole-grain oats produced by a wetting and rolling process. They are thicker and chewier than rolled oats.

**Oat Bran** — Part of the crushed oat grain left after milling. Not only bran but 3-4 layers of cells called aleurone layers.

**Oat Flour** — Finely ground oats for baking, light in texture. Make easily by grinding small amounts of rolled oats in blender.

**Quick Cooking or Rolled Oats** — Made from small whole grain oats steamed to pre-cook the flakes and then flattened to very thin flakes for quick cooking.

*OATMEAL BROTH* — To be used in creamy soups and stews as a thickener.

Combine 1 quart water and 1 cup oats. Soak overnight, then strain through a sieve. Discard oats.

## *QUINOA* (keen´-wa)

Quinoa is a grain from the Andean mountain regions of South America. Its origins are truly ancient. Along with corn and potatoes, it was a staple food of the Inca civilization, and is known as the "mother grain." Quinoa contains more protein than any other grain, an average of 16%, compared to 14% for wheat, 9.9% for millet, and 7.5% for rice. Some varieties of quinoa are over 20% protein. This protein is a complete protein, with essential amino acid balance close to ideal; it is also high in lysine, methionine, and cystine. This makes quinoa an excellent food to combine with other grains which may be low in lysine or methionine to increase protein values.

Quinoa also provides fiber, oil (it is high in linoleic acid), minerals, vitamins, starch, and sugar. Quinoa is versatile and satisfying, yet light and easily digestible. A little goes a long way. Cooked quinoa expands almost 5 times, compared to about 3 times for brown rice. That adds up to over 12 servings per pound.

**Quinoa Grain** (berries) — Simmered berries can be eaten as a cereal, added to breads, used in salads, or as a rice substitute, in casseroles, or toasted.

**Quinoa Flour** — Gluten-free. If added to favorite bread recipes (10%) it will yield a more nutritious and lighter loaf.

# RYE

Rye has a strong, hearty flavor which is great in breads and cereals. It provides protein, B-complex vitamins, calcium, iron, magnesium, phosphorus, and potassium. Dark rye flour is higher in protein, vitamins, and minerals than light rye flour.

**Whole Rye Grain** (berries) — Can be sprouted, cooked, and used as a cereal or in breads, or soaked and used in a variety of recipes like meat loaf or stuffing.

**Rye Flakes** — Berries that have been steamed and rolled, similar to oat or wheat flakes. Use in breads, cereals, and granolas.

**Rye Meal** — Coarsely ground grain that can be added to wheat flour and used in baking.

**Rye Flour** — Contains less gluten than wheat flour. Large amounts of rye flour tend to produce a sticky dough. 10-15% rye flour mixed with other flavors gives more smoothness and workability to the dough. Rye flours may vary in color depending on the variety of grain and the amount of bran left in the flour.

# TRITICALE *(trit-uh-kay´-lee)*

A grain obtained by crossing wheat with rye. It has the nutritional qualities of rye and baking qualities of wheat. Triticale is higher in the amino acid lysine, the main limiting amino acid in wheat or rye. It is also higher in protein than either wheat or rye. Triticale has a delicious, nutty flavor.

**Triticale Grain** (berries) — *To cook:* 2 parts water/1 part berries. Cover and simmer about 1 hour. To cut cooking time in half, soak overnight.

**Triticale Flour** — Has less gluten than wheat flour. Use combined with other flours, or alone in breads, pancakes, or pie crust.

# WHEAT

Whole wheat provides protein, B-complex vitamins, vitamin E, phosphorus, potassium, calcium, carbohydrate, fiber, niacin, thiamine, pyridoxine, and pantothenic acid, with traces of many other minerals. Wheat has a wonderful aroma and a distinctive nutlike flavor. It ranks with meat and dairy products as a main source of nourishment, and is by far the most popular grain in North America. The 3 most common types of wheat are:

*Hard Fall or Spring* — Stone-ground or unbleached white flours. Hard wheat is usually red, but sometimes white, and high in gluten. Used in yeast breads and cakes.

*Soft Red Winter* — Whole wheat pastry flour, unbleached white pastry flour. It has a low gluten yield, not a good choice for yeast breads, but perfect for pie crust, pancakes, and waffles. Soft wheat is a great substitute for cake flour; it gives more texture.

*Durum* — Used mostly in pastas.

The wheat grain or berry has 3 parts: The bran, or outer layer; the germ, or embryo of the grain; and the endosperm, or starchy middle part. Wheat is milled by methods that separate the grain parts, producing products such as:

**Wheat Berries** (wheat grains) — Soaked or cooked wheat berries can be used in pilafs, cereals, breads, soups, or even sprouted and tossed in a salad.

**Cracked Wheat** — Whole grains of wheat, steel cut into coarse pieces. Ideal for hot cereal, breads, and soups. Cracked wheat contains all the nutrients of the whole grain.

**Rolled Wheat** — Grains that are steamed and flattened.

**Wheat Bran** — The outer part of the grain — a valuable fiber.

**Wheat Germ** — The embryo of the grain, usually removed to prevent wheat flour from spoiling. Wheat germ provides unsaturated fat, protein, calcium, iron, phosphorus, and vitamins B and E. Keep wheat germ refrigerated to prevent its oil content from spoiling, or freeze if you wish to keep for a long period of time. Wheat germ can be eaten alone, or added to breads, cookies, casseroles, pie crusts, breading for poultry and fish, and even stirred into fresh juice. Start adding wheat germ to your diet by replacing $1/4$ cup of the flour with an equal amount of wheat germ in some of your favorite recipes.

**Wheat Sprouts** — Soak berries in a jar overnight, drain, cover with a screen. Rinse 2-3 times a day. Harvest when sprout is about as long as the berry. Use in salads, breads, even fresh juice.

**Whole Wheat Flour** — Contains the whole wheat: Bran, germ, and endosperm. Wheat flour contains the highest amount of gluten, which is the substance that gives dough its elasticity. As an added plus, it also has a hearty wheat flavor.

Whole wheat flour can be substituted for white flour, but if you are using coarse ground whole wheat flour, use about $1/4$ - $1/3$ cup less flour and, depending on the recipe and dryness, add a bit more liquid. Experiment and change your favorite recipes into favorite nutritious recipes.

**Graham Flour** — Usually the term graham flour is used interchangeably with whole wheat. Graham flour has the coarsest bran sifted out, which produces a fine caramel-colored flour, with only a bit more bran than unbleached white flour.

**Unbleached White Flour** — Is processed by huge rollers and consists of 70% of the wheat grain, the primary endosperm which is mainly STARCH. Unbleached white flour has no fiber, and contains

---

### *DO YOU HAVE WHEAT ALLERGIES?*

Substitutes for 1 cup of whole wheat flour:

| | |
|---|---|
| Barley flour | 1-1$1/2$ cups |
| Cornmeal (coarse) | $3/4$ cups |
| Oat flour | $1/4$-$1/2$ cup |
| Potato flour | $3/4$-1 cup |
| Rice flour | $3/4$-1 cup |
| Rye flour | $3/4$-1$1/4$ cups |

Add carefully, amounts may vary.

To thicken gravies, sauces, or puddings, substitute one of the following for 1 Tablespoon wheat flour:

$1/2$ Tablespoon arrowroot starch
$1/2$ Tablespoon potato starch
$1/2$ Tablespoon rice starch
$1/2$ Tablespoon tapioca

---

only 20-25% of whole wheat's vitamins and minerals. Gives lightness and increased workability to yeast breads. The bleaching process removes even more vitamins.

## OTHER FLOURS

**Potato Flour** — Gluten-free. Potatoes are steamed, dried and ground, or the starch is extracted by pulverizing and washing, to make various products, one of them being potato starch or flour. This flour has a mild flavor and expands more than other flours.

**Semolina Flour** — This term originally applied to durum wheat, but now may refer to any very coarse flour (e.g., rice semolina, corn semolina). If unqualified it means semolina from wheat. Semolina differs from other flour, which is much finer, in that when cooked it has a texture more like porridge than paste. This makes for added lightness in many dishes.

**Tapioca Flour** — Gluten-free. A slightly sweet, starchy powder-like flour derived from the cassava root. Tapioca flour is tasty added to rice or millet flours.

**Self-Rising Flour** — Flour with chemical leaveners mixed in at the mills.

**Cake Flour** — Specially treated flours that are snow white, low in gluten, starchy, soft, and finely ground. When combined with specially emulsified fat, they take up high quantities of liquid and sugar, making cakes sweet and moist.

# RAISIN BRAN BREAD — NO EGGS   3 loaves

1½ cups water
1 cup raisins
⅓ cup lukewarm water
1 package dry yeast
1 teaspoon brown sugar
2 cups 2% milk
¼ cup margarine
½ cup molasses
3-4 cups unbleached white flour
1½ cups bran
1 cup whole wheat flour

Preheat oven to 350°
In a saucepan, combine 1½ cups water and raisins; simmer until raisins are plump, about 15 minutes. Drain and save 1 cup of raisin water, then continue to drain raisins thoroughly. In a bowl, combine ⅓ cup lukewarm water, yeast, and brown sugar. Let sit about 15 minutes. In a saucepan, combine milk, margarine, molasses, and reserved raisin water. Heat until margarine melts, remove from heat, and cool. When cool, add milk mixture to yeast mixture. Stir in 1½ cups white flour and mix well. Add bran, whole wheat flour, and raisins, mixing well after each addition. Add remaining white flour. Mix well. Turn dough out onto a lightly floured surface and knead 8-10 minutes, or until dough is smooth and elastic. Place in an oiled bowl, cover with damp cloth and let rise until double in bulk, about 1 hour. Punch down once in center and turn out onto a lightly floured surface. Divide into 3 sections, knead a few times into desired loaf shapes, or rolls. Put in a warm place and let rise until double, about 35 minutes. Bake loaves for 25-30 minutes, or rolls at 400° for 8-10 minutes.

# AMARANTH SEED-BROWN RICE FLOUR BREAD — NO EGGS

2 loaves

*1 cup water*
*¼ cup amaranth seeds*
*1 package dry yeast*
*⅓ cup lukewarm water*
*1½ cups nonfat or 2% milk*
*3 Tablespoons margarine*
*½ cup molasses*
*2 cups unbleached white flour*
*1½ cups brown rice flour*

Preheat oven to 350°

In a saucepan, bring 1 cup water to boil. Add amaranth seeds and simmer on low heat for 15 minutes. Remove from heat and set aside. In a bowl, combine yeast and ⅓ cup lukewarm water. Let sit 15 minutes. In a saucepan, combine milk, margarine and molasses. Heat until margarine melts. Remove from heat and let cool. Add cooked amaranth seed and cooled milk mixture to yeast mixture and mix well. Add white flour and mix well. Add brown rice flour and mix well. Turn out onto a lightly floured surface and knead for 8-10 minutes, or until dough is smooth and elastic. Place in an oiled bowl, cover, and let rise in a warm place until double in bulk, about 1 hour. Punch dough down once in center and turn out onto a lightly floured surface. Divide into 2, and knead each slightly to form loaf. Let rise until double, about 45 minutes. Bake for 25-30 minutes.

# QUINOA AND AMARANTH
# RYE BREAD — NO EGGS

2 loaves

1 cup water
1/4 cup quinoa seeds
1/4 cup amaranth seeds
1/4 cup lukewarm water
1 package dry yeast
Pinch of sugar
1 1/2 teaspoons caraway seeds — optional
1/2 cup molasses
2 Tablespoons margarine
1 1/2 cups boiling water
3-3 1/2 cups unbleached white flour
1-1 1/2 cups rye flour

Preheat oven to 350°

In a saucepan, bring 1 cup of water to boil. Add quinoa and amaranth seeds, lower heat and simmer 15 minutes. Remove from heat and set aside. In a bowl, combine 1/4 cup lukewarm water, yeast, and pinch of sugar. Let stand at least 15 minutes. In a large bowl, combine caraway seeds, molasses, margarine, and 1 1/2 cups boiling water. Mix well and let cool. Add quinoa and amaranth seeds and yeast mixture to molasses mixture. Add 2 cups unbleached white flour and mix well. Add rye flour and mix well. Turn out onto a floured board and knead in remaining white flour until dough is smooth and elastic (about 5 minutes). Place in oiled bowl and let rise in warm place until double, about 45 minutes. Punch dough down once in center and turn out onto a lightly floured surface. Divide dough in half and shape into loaves. Let rise another 30 minutes. Bake for 30 minutes.

# AMARANTH BREAD — NO EGGS  2 loaves

*³/₄ cup molasses*
*1¹/₂ cups rye flakes*
*2¹/₄ cups boiling water*
*¹/₂ cup bran*
*2 Tablespoons caraway seeds*
*1 package dry yeast*
*¹/₃ cup warm water*
*Pinch of sugar*
*3 cups unbleached white flour*
*1 cup amaranth flour*

Preheat oven to 350°

In mixer, using bread hook, combine molasses, rye flakes, boiling water, bran, and caraway seeds. Soak for 1 hour. (If you get busy and can't get back to it, don't panic. This mixture can sit overnight.) In a small bowl, combine yeast, warm water, and a pinch of sugar, and set aside for 15 minutes.

Combine yeast mixture and molasses mixture and mix well. Add half the flour and mix well, then add remaining flour and mix well again. Turn out onto a lightly floured board and knead until dough forms a smooth, elastic ball. Place in an oiled bowl and cover. Let rise 1 hour in warm place or until double in size. Punch down, shape into desired loaves or rolls and let rise for another 30 minutes. Bake for 30-35 minutes. Bake rolls at 400° for 8-10 minutes.

# BROWN RICE RAISIN BREAD

4 loaves

1½ cups water
1 cup raisins
⅓ cup lukewarm water
2 packages dry yeast
¼ teaspoon sugar
⅓ cup soybean margarine
1 cup nonfat milk
½ cup molasses
2 eggs
1½ cups brown rice flour
1 cup whole wheat flour
1 cup bran
2½-3½ cups unbleached white flour

Preheat oven to 350°

In a saucepan, combine 1½ cups water and 1 cup raisins, simmer until raisins are plump, drain off 1 cup of raisin water, and set aside for later use, continuing to drain raisins.

In a bread bowl, combine ⅓ cup lukewarm water, yeast, and sugar. Let sit for 15 minutes.

Meanwhile, in a saucepan combine margarine, milk, molasses, and raisin water. Heat until margarine melts, remove from heat, and let cool.

Beat eggs and stir into yeast mixture. Add cooled milk mixture and mix well.

Combine brown rice flour, whole wheat flour, bran, and 2½ cups white flour. (Set aside 1 cup white flour for kneading.)

Add half of flour mixture to yeast and milk mixture, mix well. Add raisins and remaining flour mixture and mix well. Turn out onto a lightly floured surface, using the reserved white flour, and knead dough about 5-8 minutes, until smooth and elastic. Place dough in an oiled bowl and cover with a damp cloth. Set in a warm place and let rise until double in bulk, about 1 hour. Punch down once in center of dough, separate into 2, let rest 5 minutes and divide dough again, for total of 4 sections. Shape into desired loaves or rolls. Let rise in warm place until double in size. Bake loaves for 30-35 minutes. Bake rolls at 400° for 8-10 minutes.

Note: For a cinnamon loaf, mix together 1 teaspoon cinnamon, $1/3$ cup brown sugar, and $1/3$ teaspoon nutmeg. Before shaping loaf, flatten dough slightly, sprinkle with cinnamon mixture, knead a couple of times to shape loaf, let rise until double, and bake as directed above.
Loaves freeze well.

# WHOLE WHEAT BREAD

4 loaves

*2 packages dry yeast*
*½ cup lukewarm water*
*1 teaspoon sugar*
*2 cups nonfat milk*
*⅓ cup margarine — try soybean margarine*
*⅓ cup molasses*
*2 eggs*
*3 cups unbleached white flour*
*2 cups whole wheat flour — medium ground*

Preheat oven to 350°

In a small bowl, combine yeast, lukewarm water, and sugar. Let sit for 15 minutes. In a saucepan, combine milk, margarine, and molasses; heat until margarine melts, remove from heat, and let cool to lukewarm. In a large bread bowl, combine lukewarm milk mixture and yeast mixture. Add 2 eggs, and mix well. Add 2 cups white flour and mix well, then add remaining white flour and 2 cups whole wheat flour and mix well again. Turn out onto a floured surface and knead for 5-10 minutes, until dough is smooth and elastic. Place in an oiled bowl, cover with a damp cloth, and set aside in a warm place. Let rise until double in bulk, about 1 hour. Punch down dough in center with 2 fingers. Turn out onto a lightly floured surface and separate into 4 sections. Let sit a minute or so, then shape each section into loaves or rolls. Cover with a towel. Let rise an additional 30-40 minutes. Bake loaves for 25-30 minutes; bake rolls at 400° for 8-10 minutes.

# FLAT BREAD

The Austrian version is made with rye flour and is hard and thick. A supply was intended to keep for many months in the snowbound mountains of Austria. We like using it for our lunches while skiing. This bread is hard and crisp. Reduce baking time for chewy version. Great dipped into soups and stews, or topped with cheese.

*1 package yeast*
*2 cups lukewarm water*
*2 cups whole wheat flour*
*¼ teaspoon salt*
*1 teaspoon fennel seed*
*2½ cups white flour*

Preheat oven to 375°

In large bowl, dissolve yeast in water. Mix whole wheat flour, salt, and fennel seed together, and add to yeast mixture. Beat until smooth. Stir in enough white flour, about 2½ cups, to form a soft dough. Turn dough onto a lightly floured surface and knead until dough is no longer sticky, adding more flour as needed. Place dough in an oiled bowl. Cover and let stand in warm place until doubled in size, approximately 45 minutes. Punch down once in center. Knead briefly to release air, and then divide into 6 equal sections. Flatten out each section on an oiled baking sheet, about 8 inches in diameter. Cover and let rise until double, about 30 minutes. Prick surface of each flat bread with a fork. Optional: Brush each with egg white.
Bake until well browned, 25-30 minutes for hard flat bread or 20 minutes for chewy flat bread.

Note: If you can't bake dough all at once, wrap and refrigerate. Shape and bake later.

# CRANBERRY BREAD I

1 large loaf

1 cup sugar
2 Tablespoons unsalted butter
1 egg, beaten
1 cup orange juice
2 cups unbleached white flour
½ teaspoon baking powder
½ teaspoon baking soda
1 cup cranberries — cut in half
½ cup walnuts — chopped

Preheat oven to 350°
Cream sugar and butter. Add egg, orange juice and mix well. In a bowl, combine flour, baking powder, baking soda and mix well. Combine dry ingredients with sugar-butter mixture, mix well. Add cranberries and nuts, mix well. Bake in well greased pan for 1 hour and 10 minutes. Cool for 10 minutes. Remove from pan. Wrap in foil and chill from 12-24 hours.

Yeast should be dissolved in warm, NOT HOT, water. Maximum temperatures are 104° for cake yeast and 115° for dry yeast. Check on your wrist to see if the water is too warm.

# CRANBERRY BREAD II
1 large or 3 small loaves

*1 egg, beaten*
*½ cup date sugar*
*½ cup turbinado or brown sugar*
*2 Tablespoons margarine, melted*
*1 cup orange juice*
*⅔ cup 2% milk*
*1 cup unbleached white flour*
*1 cup whole wheat flour*
*½ teaspoon baking soda*
*½ teaspoon baking powder*
*⅓ cup unsalted sunflower seeds*
*1 cup cranberries — cut in halves or quarters*

Preheat oven to 350°
In a bowl, combine beaten egg with sugars and margarine. Mix well. Add orange juice and milk, and set aside. In another bowl, mix dry ingredients: White flour, wheat flour, baking soda, baking powder, and sunflower seeds. Combine wet and dry ingredients and fold in cranberries. In a well greased and floured pan, bake 1 hour and 10 minutes, or in 3 small pans for 40 minutes. Cool 10 minutes before removing from pan. Best when refrigerated for 24 hours before serving.

Tip: Freeze cranberries, then cut in half with kitchen knife.

# BROCCOLI TOFU BREAD — NO EGGS

1 large loaf

*½ cup soybean margarine or unsalted butter*
*¾ cup sugar*
*1 cup cooked broccoli — chopped fine*
*1 cup plain tofu — drained and chopped*
*1 teaspoon baking soda*
*2½ teaspoons dried sweet basil*
*1 cup whole wheat flour*
*½ cup soya flour*
*½ cup unbleached white flour*
*¾ cup buttermilk or ½ cup canned milk with 2 teaspoons of vinegar*

Preheat oven to 350°

Cream margarine and sugar, add broccoli and tofu, soda, basil, and flours. Slowly add buttermilk. Pour into greased and floured bread pan. Bake 45 minutes to 1 hour. Check for doneness with toothpick.

# CHEWY GRANOLA-DRIED APPLE MUFFINS

1 dozen large muffins

*½ cup granola*
*½ cup bran*
*¾ cup whole wheat flour*
*¼ cup unbleached white flour*
*½ cup dried apples — chopped*
*1 Tablespoon baking powder*
*1 egg*
*½ cup buttermilk*
*3 Tablespoons sunflower or safflower oil*

260

*½ cup boiling water*
*½ cup molasses*

Preheat oven to 350°

In a bowl, mix granola, bran, flours, apples, and baking powder. In another bowl combine egg, buttermilk, and oil. Mix boiling water and molasses. Mix all ingredients together. Bake in greased and floured muffin tins for 20-25 minutes. Be sure to check muffins as not all ovens are the same temperature.

# CORNMEAL AND DRIED APPLE MUFFINS

1 dozen large muffins

*1 cup cornmeal*
*1 cup dried apples — chopped*
*½ cup walnuts — chopped*
*¾ cup whole wheat flour*
*¼ cup unbleached white flour*
*1 teaspoon baking powder*
*¾ cup hot water*
*¾ cup molasses*
*1 egg — beaten*
*1 teaspoon oil*

Preheat oven to 375°

Mix dry ingredients in bowl and set aside. In bowl, mix hot water and molasses. Add beaten egg and oil. Add dry ingredients. Bake in greased and floured muffin tins for 20 minutes.

## WHOLE WHEAT BLUEBERRY MUFFINS

1 dozen

*½ cup unbleached white flour*
*½ cup whole wheat flour — medium ground*
*¼ cup bran*
*2 teaspoons baking powder*
*¾ cup walnuts — chopped*
*1 egg*
*½ cup molasses*
*⅓ cup oil — I use polyunsaturated safflower oil*
*1 cup fresh blueberries — drain if using canned*

Preheat oven to 400°

In a bowl, combine white flour, whole wheat flour, bran, baking powder, and walnuts. Mix. With spoon make a well in the center of flour mixture.

In another bowl, beat egg. Add molasses and oil to egg and mix well. Pour egg mixture into well in flour. Mix until blended. Fold in blueberries, stirring lightly. Fill oiled muffin tins and bake for 20-25 minutes.

## BLUEBERRY MUFFINS

1 dozen

*1 cup unbleached white flour*
*¾ cup brown rice flour*
*1½ teaspoons baking powder*
*¼ cup brown sugar*
*1 egg*
*⅔ cup buttermilk*
*¼ cup oil*

*Pinch of salt — optional*
*1 cup fresh blueberries*

Preheat oven to 400°

Combine flours, baking powder, and brown sugar. Make a well in center. In a small bowl, combine egg, buttermilk, oil, and salt. Add all at once to dry ingredients. Stir quickly just until dry ingredients are moistened. Add washed blueberries. Gently fold into batter. Fill greased muffin pan ⅔ full. Bake about 25 minutes.

---

# MARY'S BLUEBERRY BARS

*1 cup walnuts — chopped*
*½ cup honey*
*¼ cup margarine*
*2 cups whole wheat flour*
*1 teaspoon baking soda*
*2 cups blueberries — washed and drained*
*2 eggs*
*1½ teaspoons cinnamon*
*⅓ cup raw wheat germ*
*1 cup buttermilk*

Preheat oven to 350°

Sprinkle a 9x13 oiled pan with chopped nuts. In a bowl, mix honey, margarine, flour, and baking soda with a fork until mixture is crumbly. Spread 2 cups of the flour mixture over the nuts, and pat smooth. Spread blueberries over top. In a mixing bowl, beat eggs. Add cinnamon, wheat germ, buttermilk, and remaining flour mixture. Pour over blueberries. Bake for 35-40 minutes. Cool and cut into bars.

# KOLACHE 86

About 1 dozen rolls

1 cup prunes, pitted and chopped
2 Tablespoons sugar
½ teaspoon cinnamon
2½ cups brown rice flour
2½ cups unbleached white flour
1 package dry yeast
⅓ cup lukewarm water
½ teaspoon sugar
1¾ cup nonfat milk — scalded
⅓ cup unsalted butter
½ cup molasses
1 egg — beaten

Preheat oven to 350°

In a saucepan, combine prunes, 2 Tablespoons sugar, and cinnamon. Add enough water to cover prunes. Simmer on low heat until prunes are tender. Mash prune mixture with fork and set aside.
In a large bowl, mix rice flour and white flour and set aside.
In a small bowl, mix together yeast, lukewarm water, and ½ teaspoon sugar. Let sit for 15 minutes.
In a saucepan, heat nonfat milk, butter, and molasses. When butter has melted, cool mixture until lukewarm, then add yeast mixture and beaten egg. Mix well. Add 2 cups flour mixture and mix well. Add 2 more cups flour mixture and mix again. Turn dough out onto a lightly floured surface and, using remaining flour, knead dough 3-5 minutes. Place into a large greased bowl, cover with a damp cloth, and set bowl in a warm place. Let rise until double in size, about 1 hour. Punch down once in center of dough. Cover bowl again, and let rise a second time. Roll out on a floured surface to about ½ inch thickness and cut into squares. Add dab of prune mixture in the center of each square. Bring up corners and pinch. Bake for 25 minutes.

# CHEERIO-DATE GRANOLA

Approximately 6 cups

*2 cups rolled oats*
*¹/₂ cup unsalted sunflower seeds*
*1 cup Cheerios*
*1¹/₂ Tablespoons oil*
*¹/₂ cup molasses*
*¹/₄ cup water*
*1 cup dates — chopped, dredged in 2 Tablespoons flour*
*1 cup unsalted cashews*
*1 cup banana chips*

Preheat oven to 275°

Mix oats, sunflower seeds, and Cheerios together on a cookie sheet. In a bowl, mix together oil, molasses, and water, mixing well. Pour over dry mixture on cookie sheet. Mix, coating everything well. Bake for ¹/₂ hour, mixing every 15 minutes. Add dates, cashews, and banana chips, and bake another ¹/₂ hour, mixing frequently. Remove from oven and let air dry at least ¹/₂ hour. Store in airtight containers.

265

# MOLASSES GRANOLA SNACK

Approximately 5$^1/_2$ cups

*1 cup rolled oats*
*1 cup rye flakes*
*1 cup 7 grain flakes*
*1 cup unsalted sunflower seeds*
*1 cup molasses*
*2 Tablespoons safflower oil*
*1 cup roasted soybeans*

Preheat oven to 250°

On a large cookie sheet, mix rolled oats, rye flakes, 7 grain flakes, and sunflower seeds.

In a bowl, mix $^2/_3$ cup molasses and oil. Mix well and pour over mixture on cookie sheet. Mix until everything is well coated. Place in oven for $^1/_2$ hour, stirring every 15 minutes. Pour remaining $^1/_3$ cup molasses over mixture and mix well. Return to oven for 45 minutes, mixing well every 15 minutes. Remove from oven and add roasted soybeans. Let dry for at least $^1/_2$ hour. Store in airtight containers. Eat as cold cereal or trail snack.

# FRIDAY THE 13TH GRANOLA

Approximately 6 cups

*1¼ cups rolled oats*
*¾ cup almonds*
*½ cup unsweetened shredded coconut*
*2 Tablespoons oil*
*¼ cup honey*
*¼ cup molasses*
*1 cup raisins*
*1 cup dates — chopped*
*2 Tablespoons flour*
*1 cup banana chips*

Preheat oven to 250°

Place oats, almonds, and coconut on a cookie sheet. In a bowl, mix oil, honey, and molasses. Pour over cookie sheet mixture and mix until well coated. Place in oven for 1 hour, mixing every 15 minutes. Remove from oven and add raisins and dates that have been dredged in flour and are well coated. Mix well. Return to oven for another 45 minutes, mixing every 15 minutes. Remove from oven and add banana chips. Return to oven for ½ hour longer, mixing frequently. Cool completely. Store in airtight containers or in your refrigerator or freezer.

# CHOCOLATE CHIP COOKIES

Approximately 4 dozen small cookies

*¾ cup whole wheat flour — medium ground*
*1 cup unbleached white flour*
*½ teaspoon baking soda*
*½ cup light margarine (or unsalted butter)*
*¼ cup brown sugar*
*⅓ cup molasses*
*2 eggs*
*1½ teaspoons vanilla*
*12-ounce bag of chocolate chips (or carob chips if desired)*
*½ cup almond slivers — optional*

Preheat oven to 350°

Mix all dry ingredients and set aside. In a bowl, cream together margarine, brown sugar, and molasses. Add eggs and vanilla, mixing well. Add half flour mixture, again mixing well. Add chocolate chips and nuts, and then remaining flour, mixing well after each addition. Drop by teaspoonfuls onto ungreased cookie sheets. Bake 5-7 minutes.

# OATMEAL-WHEATENA COOKIES

Approximately 3½ dozen cookies

1 cup water
1 cup raisins
¾ cup soybean margarine (or unsalted butter)
1 cup sugar
2 eggs
1 teaspoon vanilla
1 cup rolled oats (not processed "quick" rolled oats)
⅓ cup Wheatena (100% toasted wheat found in the cereal section)
1 cup unbleached white flour
1 cup whole wheat flour
½ teaspoon baking soda
½ teaspoon baking powder
Dash of salt — optional
1 teaspoon cinnamon
½ teaspoon cloves
1 cup 7 grain flakes

Preheat oven to 325°

Simmer 1 cup raisins in 1 cup water until raisins are plump, about 10 minutes. In a bowl, cream together the margarine and sugar. Add eggs and vanilla. Stir in 1 cup liquid from raisins (add tap water to make one cup if needed); set aside. Mix dry ingredients and combine with egg mixture. Add raisins and mix well. Drop onto ungreased cookie sheets with a teaspoon. Bake for 10-12 minutes.

# FOR 9-INCH ONE-CRUST PIE

*1 cup unbleached white flour*
*Pinch of salt*
*⅓ cup vegetable shortening*
*2-4 Tablespoons water*

In a bowl, mix flour and salt. Cut in shortening with fork or by hand until particles are the size of peas. Sprinkle with water, 1 Tablespoon at a time, mixing with a fork, until flour is moistened. Gather dough together with fingers, press into a ball. Let dough sit for a couple of minutes. Roll out crust on a lightly floured surface, roll from center out to not quite ⅛ inch thick. Roll lightly, being careful not to add extra flour as this will toughen crust. Roll about 1 inch larger all around than pie pan. Fold crust in half. Carefully transfer to pie pan.

For baked pie shell, prick pie shell with fork and bake at 475° 8-10 minutes, or until golden brown.

# BROWN RICE PUDDING

4 servings

*1 cup water*
*³/₄ cup brown rice — rinsed*
*1 egg*
*³/₄ cup nonfat milk*
*¹/₄ cup half-and-half*
*1 cup raisins*
*¹/₂ teaspoon cinnamon*

In a saucepan, bring water to boil. Add rice and return to a boil. Reduce heat to low. Cover and let cook 30 minutes. In a bowl, beat egg. Add milk, half-and-half, raisins, and cinnamon. Add this egg mixture to rice, mix well, and simmer on low heat for 20 minutes longer. Remove from heat and let sit a few minutes before serving. Also delicious served chilled.

# MIXED RICE

4 servings

*1¹/₂ cups boiling water*
*¹/₄ cup brown rice — rinsed*
*¹/₄ cup basmati rice — rinsed*
*2 Tablespoons leeks — chopped*
*¹/₂-1 teaspoon curry powder. (If you are not used to using this spice, use only ¹/₂ teaspoon. If you like the taste of curry, use 1 teaspoon.)*

Bring water to boil. Add brown rice, basmati rice, leeks, and curry. Bring to boil and let boil 1-2 minutes. Reduce heat to low and cover. Simmer for 35-40 minutes.

## ORANGE RAISIN RICE

4 servings

1½ *cups water*
¾ *cup basmati rice — rinsed*
⅓ *cup fresh orange — peeled, sectioned and chopped*
¼ *cup raisins*

In a saucepan, bring water to a boil. Add rice, orange, and raisins. Return to a boil. Let cook 1 minute. Cover and lower heat to low. Let simmer 25-30 minutes. (Time may vary by a few minutes depending on heat source and pan being used.)

## SAFFRON RICE

4 servings

¼ *teaspoon saffron threads*
1¼ *cups water*
¼ *cup fresh mushrooms — chopped*
½ *cup basmati rice — rinsed*
2 *Tablespoons green onion — chopped*

In a small bowl, soak saffron in ¼ cup water. In a saucepan, bring 1 cup water to a boil. Add soaked saffron (with water), mushrooms, rice, and green onion. Return to a boil, cover. Cook 30-35 minutes on low heat.

# BASMATI RICE WITH TOMATOES 4 servings

*1 cup water*
*1 cup stewed tomatoes*
*½ cup fresh mushrooms — chopped*
*½ cup green onion — chopped*
*1 Tablespoon red chili sauce*
*½ cup basmati rice — rinsed*

Combine water and stewed tomatoes and bring to boil. Add mushrooms, green onions, chili sauce, and rice. Return to boil. Reduce heat to low and simmer for 30-35 minutes.

---

# NUTMEG RICE 4 servings

*2 cups water*
*½ cup basmati rice — rinsed*
*½ cup brown rice — rinsed*
*½ teaspoon ground nutmeg*

Bring water to a boil. Add basmati and brown rice. Return to boil. Add nutmeg. Lower heat to low, cover and simmer 25-30 minutes. Great served with chicken or served cold with raisins and milk.

## BREAKFAST CEREALS

Before you open that box, read the label! You may be having breakfast with a loser. Instead of eating the same boring breakfast cereal from a familiar box every morning, try creating your own cereal, hot or cold. You'll be providing your family and yourself with vitamins, minerals, and protein without the added salt, sugar, fat (added oil), and preservatives in most boxed cereals. Cereal is simple, fast, and fun to make. When made in large batches, it is as convenient to store and serve as boxed cereal.

The basic ingredient is oats, instant or non-instant, with wheat or oat bran added. Then add one or more of the following: Rye, wheat, triticale, barley flakes, quinoa, wheat germ, and 7 grain cereal, all of which should be available at your market or co-op. Sweeteners can range from honey, molasses, raisins, fresh or dried fruit, white or brown sugar (if used in limited amounts). If you like crunch, add chopped nuts, unsalted sunflower seeds, or sesame seeds. For added flavor, try cinnamon or nutmeg. Be creative and experiment with different combinations. Start enjoying the taste, texture, and health benefits of your breakfast.

The American Institute for Cancer Research suggested recipe yields 11 cups. Make ahead and serve hot or cold.

*2 cups oats*
*1 cup rye flakes*
*2 cups wheat germ*
*2 cups wheat bran*
*1 cup dates — chopped*
*½ cup almonds — slivered*
*1 cup dried fruit*
*1 teaspoon cinnamon*

To make cereal, put all ingredients in the food processor in batches and process briefly. Small amounts of cinnamon, nutmeg, and ground cloves are delicious. For special flavor, add a vanilla bean to the container in which you store your cereal. In the morning, just put some in a bowl, add milk, and savor a healthy homemade breakfast. Store in airtight containers in your pantry, refrigerator, or even in your freezer.

Use this recipe as the basic cereal and substitute different items like oat bran, wheat flakes, molasses, honey. You'll be surprised at the delicious combinations you have created. Fresh fruit is great added at serving time.

*Source: American Institute of Cancer Research Newsletter, Issue 14, Winter 1986*

# Comparison of Some Common Breakfast Cereals

These are just a sampling of the many available, but give an idea of the variety of contents. See how your cereals compare.

| Cereal | Dietary Fiber* (gm) | Sugar* (gm)** | Fat* (gm) | Sodium* (mg) | Protein* (gm) | Calories* |
|---|---|---|---|---|---|---|
| All-Bran | 9 | 5 | 1 | 270 | 4 | 70 |
| Bran Chex | 5 | 5 | 0 | 300 | 3 | 90 |
| Bran Flakes | 4-5 | 5 | 0 | 220-230 | 3 | 90 |
| Cheerios | 2 | 1 | 2 | 330 | 4 | 110 |
| Corn Bran | 5 | 6 | 1 | 300 | 2 | 120 |
| Corn Flakes | trace | 2 | 0 | 280 | 2 | 110 |
| Fiber One | 12 | 2 | 1 | 220 | 3 | 60 |
| Frosted Flakes | trace | 11 | 0 | 190 | 1 | 110 |
| Frosted Mini-Wheats | 3 | 6 | 0 | 5 | 3 | 100 |
| Grape-Nuts | 2 | 3 | 0 | 190 | 3 | 110 |
| Life | 1 | 6 | 2 | 180 | 5 | 120 |
| 100% Natural | trace | 6 | 6 | 15 | 4 | 140 |
| Product 19 | trace | 3 | 0 | 290 | 2 | 110 |
| Shredded Wheat | 3 | 0 | 1 | trace | 2 | 110 |
| Shredded Wheat 'N Bran | 4 | 0 | 1 | 0 | 3 | 110 |
| Special K | trace | 3 | 0 | 230 | 6 | 110 |
| Wheaties | 2 | 3 | 1 | 370 | 3 | 110 |

*Represents content per ounce
**4 grams of sugar = 1 teaspoon of sugar

*Source: American Institute for Cancer Research*

# OATS FOR TWO

*1¹/₂ cups water*
*¹/₂ cup rolled oats*
*¹/₄ cup oat bran*
*¹/₄ cup raisins*

In a saucepan, bring water to a boil. Add rolled oats, oat bran, and raisins. Return to boil and cook for 2 minutes, stirring constantly. Remove from heat, cover, and let sit about 3-5 minutes. Great served with milk and fresh fruit.

# OAT-BARLEY FLAKES CEREAL    4 servings

*1¹/₂ cups water*
*³/₄ cup oat flakes*
*¹/₄ cup barley flakes*
*¹/₄ teaspoon cinnamon*
*¹/₃ cup raisins*

In a saucepan, bring water to a boil. Add all ingredients, return to a boil, lower heat, and cook 3-5 minutes. Remove from heat, cover, and let sit 2-3 minutes. Serve with milk and favorite topping.

## ROLLED OATS-OAT BRAN CEREAL

3-4 servings

*1½ cups water*
*¾ cup rolled oats*
*3 Tablespoons oat bran*
*3 Tablespoons raisins*

In a saucepan, bring water to a boil. Add all ingredients, return to a boil, lower heat, and cook 2-3 minutes. Remove from heat, cover, and let sit for 1-2 minutes before serving.

## 7 GRAIN CEREAL-TRITICALE FLAKES-BRAN

3-4 servings

*¼ cup 7 grain cereal*
*¼ cup triticale flakes*
*3 Tablespoons oat bran*
*1½ Tablespoons wheat bran*
*1 cup water*
*¼ cup nonfat milk*

Place all ingredients in a saucepan. Bring to a boil, let cook 1-2 minutes. Lower heat, cover, and simmer 5-8 minutes. Garnish as you would any hot cereal.

# SCOTTISH OATS

3 servings

*½ cup "steel-cut" oats (sometimes called Scotch Oats)*
*2 Tablespoons oat bran*
*2 Tablespoons wheat bran*
*1 cup water*

In a saucepan, combine all ingredients and bring to a boil. Let boil
2 minutes, lower heat, cover, and cook about 15 minutes.
To cut down on cooking time, soak oats overnight. After bringing
to a boil, lower heat and cook only 5 minutes.

# 7 GRAIN FLAKES-TRITICALE FLAKES

3-4 servings

*1½ cups water*
*½ cup 7 grain flakes*
*¼ cup triticale flakes*

In a saucepan, bring water to a boil. Add flakes, and return to a boil.
Cook for 2-3 minutes, stirring occasionally. Remove from heat,
cover, and let sit a minute or so before serving.

## BASIC QUINOA

Yields 2 cups

*½ cup quinoa*
*1 cup water or broth*
*Pinch of sea salt*

Rinse grain several times with fresh water. Place in saucepan with water and sea salt. Bring to a boil. Cover, lower heat, and simmer 15-20 minutes or until water is absorbed. Can be used in a variety of recipes, as a cereal, or as a rice substitute.

## TOASTED QUINOA

Yields 1 cup

Rinse quinoa with fresh water. Place quinoa in a skillet (10-12 inches) over medium heat. Cook, stirring occasionally, until quinoa dries and turns a golden brown (about 15 minutes). Remove from skillet and let cool. Store in airtight container in cool place.

## MIXED CEREAL

3 servings

*½ cup oatmeal*
*½ cup 7 grain cereal*
*1 Tablespoon oat bran*
*¼ cup nonfat milk*
*¾ cup water*

In a saucepan, combine all ingredients and bring to a boil. Reduce heat, cover, and simmer for 8-10 minutes.

# PASTA

Fresh pasta is a real treat for the whole family. It is nutritious, inexpensive, easy, delicious, and fun to make. A great project for a rainy day while listening to your favorite music, or a special project to do with your child. Even my husband likes to get involved with the rolling and cutting. Pasta is also great for the working person because with very little time or effort, you can make enough for the work week ahead.

**By Hand** — Heap flour on a floured surface, make a well in the center, place eggs, oil and any remaining ingredients into the well. With a fork, combine egg mixture and gradually mix in flour, adding water a Tablespoon at a time until dough forms a ball. Do not let dough become too sticky. Knead dough 2-3 minutes and divide into 5 or 6 small balls. Dough can sit chilled up to 3 hours. Just let stand at room temperature for half an hour before rolling.

**With Food Processor** — Combine all ingredients except water. Add water a Tablespoon at a time until ball is formed. Dough should be firm, not sticky. Blend 10-15 seconds longer to knead. Dough may be chilled up to 3 hours. Let stand half an hour at room temperature before rolling.

**Rolling** — Set the smooth roller at its lowest number. Rollers will be wide apart. Take a small ball of dough, flatten slightly with hand and dust with flour. Feed it through the rollers, fold in half and feed through rollers again. Repeat about 10 times, folding dough in half each time. Dust with flour when needed to prevent dough from sticking. Turn dial up 1 notch and roll dough through without folding over. Continue rolling dough through each notch 1 time until desired thickness. For thin pasta continue through notch 6. Dough should now be a long, smooth sheet about 4-5 inches wide. Roll through cutter. Hang to dry. You can use pasta drying racks, clothes hanger with a dish towel draped over it, or even the back of a kitchen chair with a dish cloth draped over it.

To start your pasta machine rolling I'll list a few of our favorite recipes and you can go from there. The variations are endless. I use unbleached white flour and whole wheat flour in the following recipes, but don't stop there. Remember also that fresh pasta is a great gift from the kitchen for friends and relatives.

## SPINACH WHOLE WHEAT PASTA Serves 6

*1½ cups unbleached white flour*
*½ cup whole wheat flour*
*Pinch of salt — optional*
*¼ cup water — add 1 Tablespoon at a time*
*2 eggs*
*2 cups raw spinach — chopped*
*1 Tablespoon olive oil*

In a saucepan, bring 1 cup water to a boil. Add chopped spinach and cook for 2-3 minutes. Drain spinach completely. Squeeze with hand to remove excess water. Mince drained spinach. Add eggs, oil and spinach into well made in center of flour. Follow directions for mixing and rolling.

# WHOLE WHEAT AND BRAN PASTA

*1 cup unbleached flour*
*$1/2$ cup bran*
*$1/2$ cup whole wheat flour*
*Pinch of salt — optional*
*2 eggs*
*1 Tablespoon olive oil*
*About $1/3$ cup water — add 1 Tablespoon at a time*

Follow mixing and rolling directions.

# PARSLEY WHOLE WHEAT PASTA

*$1^1/2$ cups unbleached white flour*
*$1/2$ cup whole wheat flour*
*2 eggs*
*2 Tablespoons olive oil*
*$1^1/2$ Tablespoons fresh parsley — chopped*
*4-5 Tablespoons water — add 1 Tablespoon at a time*

Follow mixing and rolling directions.

# GARLIC OREGANO PASTA

1½ *cups unbleached white flour*
½ *cup whole wheat flour*
¼ *head of garlic — blanched and mashed*
2 *Tablespoons dried oregano*
*Pinch of salt — optional*
2 *eggs*
1 *Tablespoon olive oil*
⅓ *cup water — add 1 Tablespoon at a time*

Refer to page 91 on how to blanch garlic.
Follow mixing and rolling directions.

# RED BELL PEPPER PASTA

1½ *cups unbleached white flour*
½ *cup whole wheat flour*
1 *cup red bell pepper — chopped*
2 *eggs*
1 *Tablespoon olive oil*
*About ⅓ cup water — add 1 Tablespoon at a time*

In a saucepan, bring 1 cup water to boil. Add chopped bell pepper, cook 2-3 minutes, remove from heat and drain. Place bell pepper in blender and purée (will make about ¼ cup purée).
Follow mixing and rolling directions.

## PASTA SIDE DISH

3-4 servings

*4 garlic cloves — diced*
*2 Tablespoons green onion — chopped*
*1 Tablespoon fresh basil — chopped*
*2 teaspoons olive oil*
*1 Tablespoon fresh lemon juice*
*8 ounces pasta — cooked and drained*
*¼ cup parmesan cheese — grated (or your favorite lowfat cheese)*

In a skillet heat oil, combine garlic, green onion, basil, and lemon juice and let sauté 1-2 minutes. Place cooked pasta in a serving bowl. Add mixture in skillet and toss. Top with cheese. This is a quick, tasty side dish.

## PASTA SIDE DISH WITH DRIED TOMATOES

4 servings

*8 ounces pasta*
*1 Tablespoon olive oil*
*2½ Tablespoons garlic — diced (about 6 cloves)*
*2 Tablespoons sun-dried tomatoes — diced*
*¾ cup nonfat milk*
*2 Tablespoons parmesan cheese — grated*
*2 Tablespoons romano cheese — grated*

In a saucepan, cook pasta in boiling water till tender. In a skillet, heat oil. Add garlic and sun-dried tomatoes. Sauté for a couple of minutes. Drain cooked pasta and add to skillet. Toss. Add milk, let cook 2-3 minutes. Place pasta into a serving dish and toss with fresh grated cheese. Serve immediately.

## BEANS

Beans have always been a favorite for their economy, but are also recognized as a valued food by the American Heart Association, American Cancer Society and American Diabetes Association, along with many other health-related groups.

Why? Because dry beans offer you a remarkable combination of qualities. They are:
- high in protein
- high in complex carbohydrates
- high in dietary fiber
- cholesterol-free
- low in fats
- low in sodium
- among the richest natural sources of the B-complex vitamins (thiamine, pyridoxine, niacin, and folic acid) and also contain many important minerals (iron, phosphorus, potassium, magnesium, and zinc).

*BEANS SUPPLY PROTEIN* — The protein in beans is called an incomplete protein because beans are low in methionine, one of the essential amino acids. However, despite the lack of this amino acid, the "incomplete" protein is easily made "complete" by serving beans with a food high in methionine, such as rice or corn. The proteins found in beans and rice or corn are said to be "complementary" proteins. Bean protein can also be made "complete" by serving beans with small amounts of meat, fish, cheese, or eggs.

*BEANS SUPPLY ENERGY* — Beans are an exceptional source of complex carbohydrates, the most efficient source of energy. Complex carbohydrates are digested and absorbed more slowly than simple carbohydrates and thus satisfy hunger over longer periods.

*BEANS SUPPLY FIBER* — One cup of cooked beans provides half the recommended daily intake of dietary fiber of 35-45 grams, as suggested by the American Institute of Cancer Research. This is

286

equivalent to the fiber in 10 slices of whole wheat bread or 3-4 cups cooked vegetables.

If all this is not enough to convince you to eat beans, another great nutritional virtue of dry beans is their ability to combine with so many other foods like salads, casseroles, soups, yellow and green vegetables, tomatoes, and even fruit, all of which make up a part of a balanced, healthful diet.

**Aduki Beans** (also spelled Adzuki) — A cousin of kidney beans, less known in North America but second in popularity only to soybeans in Japan. Aduki beans have a distinctive "less beany" flavor. Dry uncooked beans can be ground into a meal and added to breads and pancakes.

**Black Beans** — Small black beans with little white dots, wonderful in soups, sauces, or as a side dish.

**Black-Eyed Peas** — Are a favorite of many, white beans with a black eye, sold dry.

**Garbanzo Beans** — Also called chick peas, sold both dried and canned. Garbanzo beans can be used in a variety of ways from spaghetti sauce to salads.

**Great Northern Beans** — Larger than the small white or navy beans, and a good bean to bake.

**Kidney Beans** — Can be light or dark red. The dark beans are usually sold in cans and are delicious in salads. The light beans are usually dried, used in soups, chili and stews.

**Lima Beans** — Also called butter beans for their creamy texture. Lima beans come in 2 sizes, baby and large. The large beans are more starchy than the smaller ones, and particularly good in soups and stews. Avoid lima beans if shells look dry, shriveled or yellow. They will have poor flavor.

**Pink Beans** — Used often in Mexican cooking and "pot" of bean dishes. Sold dried or canned.

**Pinto Beans** — Colorful pink with maroon patterning. Popular in chili, refried beans, and other Mexican treats.

**Red Beans** — Dark red, pea-shaped. Use in any colored bean recipe.

**Small White Beans** (Navy Beans) — Used to make Boston baked beans, have a firm texture and hold up well under long, slow baking.

**Soybeans** — Medium-sized beans, creamy yellow in color. Also available are black soybeans imported from China. Soybeans are very versatile, can be eaten cooked, sprouted, steamed, or ground into flour for baking, or cracked into grits for cereal.

**Split Peas** — Small peas, similar to lentils. Come in green or yellow.

## HOW TO PREPARE

There are several ways to prepare dry beans for cooking and all start with a thorough checking for foreign materials or damaged beans. Then wash the beans in cold water. Soaking is not absolutely essential. However, some methods of soaking shorten cooking time, along with improving digestibility, texture and flavor.

*Overnight Soaking* — Use 6-10 cups of water per pound of beans and let soak overnight in refrigerator or a cool place. Drain and rinse.

*Preferred Method* — Bring 6-10 cups water to a boil, add beans and cook 2-3 minutes, remove from heat, cover, and soak 4-12 hours.

*Quick Method* — Bring 6-10 cups water to boil per pound of beans. Add beans and boil 2-3 minutes, remove from heat, and soak 1 hour.

After soaking, discard the "soak" water. Rinse beans and cook in fresh water. Remember to use a large enough pan for soaking because beans expand.

*Cooking* — Place beans in a pot with fresh water to cover. Bring to a boil, and let simmer on medium to medium-low heat until beans are tender. Check them occasionally and add more water if needed. It is important that beans are covered with liquid at all times. For added flavor, add ½ cup chopped onions and 1 or 2 cloves of garlic while beans are cooking. Once beans are tender they are ready to eat immediately, or you can use them in your favorite recipe, or store them for future use. Various beans differ slightly in their nutritional profile, so it is a good idea to eat a variety of beans.

Note: At high altitudes, beans take longer to cook. A pressure cooker helps shorten cooking time. Be sure to follow manufacturer's directions.

If using hard water add ¹/₈ teaspoon baking soda to shorten cooking time.

*Storage* — Keep beans in airtight containers and store in cupboard or pantry. Store leftovers in the refrigerator for a day or 2. If beans are to be used at a later time, simply store in containers and freeze.

*DIGESTIBILITY OF BEANS* — Beans contain 2 unusual starches, trisaccharides (specifically raffinase and stachyose), which are not easily broken down by the intestinal enzymes. These starches break down slowly and are believed to form gastrointestinal gas. Beans are very digestible but the flatulence (gas) discourages some people from eating them. A couple of ways to help alleviate the gas are: Soak the beans, discard the water, add fresh water and simmer for half an hour, discard the water, add fresh water, and then continue with your recipe. Another way is to add beans to your diet, gradually starting with light portions and building up, or starting with bean sprouts.

# HOW LONG TO COOK BEANS

Time on cooking chart represents approximate times for cooking beans after soaking.

| 1 CUP SOAKED | WATER | TIME | YIELDS | PRESSURE COOKER WATER | TIME (minutes) |
|---|---|---|---|---|---|
| Aduki Beans | 3 cups | 3 hours | | to cover | 20 |
| Black Beans | 4 cups | 1½ hours | 2 cups | to cover | 20 |
| Black-Eyed Peas | 3 cups | 1 hour | 2 cups | to cover | 20 |
| Garbanzo Beans or Chick Peas | 4 cups | 2-2½ hours | 2 cups | to cover | 25 |
| Great Northern Beans | 3½ cups | 1½-2 hours | 2 cups | to cover | 20 |
| Kidney Beans | 3 cups | 1-1½ hours | 2 cups | to cover | 20 |
| Lentils | 3 cups | 35 minutes | 2¼ cups | to cover | 10 |
| Lima Beans | | | | | |
|     Large | 3 cups | 1½ hours | 1¼ cups | to cover | 15 |
|     Small | 3 cups | 1¾ hours | | to cover | 10 |
| Pink Beans | 3 cups | 1 hour | 2 cups | to cover | 20 |
| Pinto Beans | 3 cups | 1½-2 hours | 2 cups | to cover | 10 |
| Red Beans | 3 cups | 2½-3 hours | 2 cups | to cover | 20 |
| Small White or Navy Beans | 3 cups | 1½ hours | 2 cups | to cover | 20 |
| Soybeans | 3 cups | 3 hours | 2 cups | to cover | 30 or more |
| Soy Grits | 2 cups | 15 minutes | 2 cups | | |
| Split Peas | 3 cups | 45 minutes | 2¼ cups | to cover | 10 |

# LENTILS

Lentils and beans are members of the same family but differ in that there are only 1 or 2 lentil seeds in each tiny pod. There are anywhere from 25-100 pods on a single plant. Naturally dried seeds are separated from the plant and pod at harvest. The seed has a skin which is removed in a process called decortication, which exposes the bright color inside the lentil and shortens cooking time. Lentils do not require soaking and the cooking time varies from 15 minutes to 1 hour. Like beans, lentils are an inexpensive source of protein.

The varieties are as follows:

**Chilean** — Green to golden brown, highly nutritious.

**Green** — Plump lentils, green to black skin with yellow interior. Also known as the petite black or dry green. Stronger flavor and firmer texture.

**Persian** — Most common variety worldwide. Smallest lentil is round, has a brown skin but after decortication is bright red. Great in salads.

**Red Chief** — Orange in color and short cooking time best describes the Red Chief lentil. The flavor is similar to Chilean lentils.

## HOW TO COOK

| | FORM | TENDER TO BITE |
|---|---|---|
| Chilean | Skin on | 30-40 minutes |
| Green | Skin on | 30-40 minutes |
| Persian | Decorticated | 15 minutes |
| | Skin on | 50-60 minutes |
| Red Chief | Decorticated | 15 minutes |
| | Skin on | 20-30 minutes |

## HOW TO PREPARE

Sort lentils and remove any rocks. Rinse and drain. Bring water to boil and add lentils, cover, simmer until tender, and drain. Use as is or add to a favorite recipe. Can be refrigerated up to 5 days. One pound of raw lentils (2¼ cups) yields 6 cups cooked. Lentils are great in soups, salads, and stews, and are all very good toasted. Use your imagination. For complete protein utilization, eat lentils with grains, nuts, seeds or dairy products. Store your lentils in airtight jars and they will keep indefinitely.

---

## *LENTIL SHRIMP SALAD* 6 servings

*¼ cup brown lentils*
*¼ cup pink lentils*
*½ cup carrots — grated*
*½ cup cabbage — shredded*
*½ cup fresh shrimp — rinsed and drained or use canned*
*2 Tablespoons lemon juice*
*¼ cup celery — chopped*
*1 teaspoon dried dill*
*Pepper to taste — optional*
*3 Tablespoons red wine vinegar*
*1 Tablespoon olive oil*
*1 Tablespoon honey*
*½ teaspoon dried marjoram*

Place lentils in saucepan with water to cover. Cook lentils on low heat for about 20 minutes or until tender, not mushy. Drain cooking water, rinse with cold water, and drain well.
In a bowl, mix lentils with all other ingredients. Toss well and chill.

# CURRIED LENTILS

4 servings

*2 cups water*
*¹/₂ cup lentils — rinsed*
*1 Tablespoon medium-strength curry powder*

In a saucepan, bring water to boil. Add rinsed lentils and curry powder. Lower heat and simmer until tender, but not mushy, about 15 minutes. Remove from heat and drain.
Use as a side dish or chilled in a salad, or as stuffing.

# LENTIL TURKEY SALAD

4-6 servings

*¹/₂ cup lentils — rinsed*
*1 cup cooked turkey — cut into bite-sized pieces*
*¹/₄ cup black olives — sliced*
*¹/₂ cup green pepper — chopped*
*¹/₂ cup onion — cut in half and sliced thin*
*2 teaspoons medium-strength curry powder*
*1 teaspoon olive oil*
*2 Tablespoons safflower mayonnaise*
*1 Tablespoon plain nonfat yogurt*

Place lentils in saucepan with water to cover. Cook lentils on low heat for about 15-20 minutes until tender but not mushy. Drain cooking water, rinse with cold water, and drain.
In a bowl, mix lentils with remaining ingredients. Toss and chill well.

# LENTILS AND HOCKS

4 servings

*2 pork hocks (about ½ pound) — trim off all excess fat*
*1 cup brown lentils — rinsed well*
*3 cups water*
*¼ cup onion — chopped*
*Pepper, to taste*

Combine all ingredients and bring to a boil. Lower heat to medium or medium-low and simmer about 2 hours. Stir occasionally.

---

# ALL-DAY POT OF BEANS

4 servings

*2 cups pinto beans — picked over and rinsed well*
*4 garlic cloves — chopped*
*2 dried red chili pods — use whole for easy removal*
*1 Tablespoon olive oil*

Combine all ingredients in a pot, with enough water to cover. Bring to a boil, lower heat, and simmer 4-5 hours. When beans are tender, remove chili pods and discard.
To shorten cooking time, soak beans overnight. Check page 288 for soaking information.

# GREAT POT OF BEANS

4-6 servings

*¼ cup kidney beans*
*¼ cup soybeans*
*¼ cup pinto beans*
*3 garlic cloves — chopped*
*4 cups of water*
*1 cup onion — chopped*
*5 fresh mushrooms — washed and quartered*
*1 cup green bell pepper — chopped*
*2 green onions — chopped*
*2 medium-sized Italian tomatoes — chopped into large chunks*
*2 bay leaves*
*1 teaspoon dried thyme*
*1 Tablespoon molasses*
*Pepper*
*1 whole chicken breast — remove skin and debone (save bones)*
*½ cup tomato sauce*

Soak beans overnight in refrigerator with water to cover.
In a kettle, combine beans, garlic, water, and onions. Simmer, covered, for 1 hour over medium heat. Add mushrooms, green bell peppers, green onions, tomatoes, bay leaves, thyme, molasses and pepper. Simmer on low heat for 1 hour. Cut chicken into bite-sized pieces. Add chicken, chicken bones, and tomato sauce and simmer over medium heat for 45 minutes. Remove bones before serving.

Note: If Italian tomatoes are not available, substitute 8 small cherry tomatoes or 2 medium tomatoes.

# CHRISTINE'S LONE STAR CAVIAR

Approximately 7¹/₂ cups

*1 pound (2 cups) dried black-eyed peas*
*2 cups Italian salad dressing*
*2 cups green peppers — diced*
*1 cup green onion — chopped fine*
*¹/₂ cup jalapeño peppers — chopped fine*
*1 - 3 ounce jar pimiento — drained*
*1 Tablespoon garlic — chopped fine*
*Salt to taste*
*Hot pepper sauce to taste (very little)*
*1¹/₂ cups onion — diced*

Soak black-eyed peas in enough water to cover for 6 hours or over-night. Drain well. Transfer peas to a saucepan. Add enough water to cover. Bring to boil over high heat. Reduce heat and simmer until peas are tender, about 45 minutes.
DO NOT OVERCOOK! Drain well, then transfer to a large bowl. Add Italian dressing and cool. (I place mixture into the refrigerator until completely cool.) Add remaining ingredients and mix well. Lone Star Caviar will vary in "hotness," depending on peppers, onions, and hot sauce. At my house, we eat Lone Star Caviar as a salad. At Christmas, it's used more as a relish or garnish.
If desired, caviar may be placed into pint jars filled to within ¹/₂ inch of top of jar. Jars should be sterilized and cooled before adding caviar. May be kept up to 10 days in the refrigerator.

# NOTES

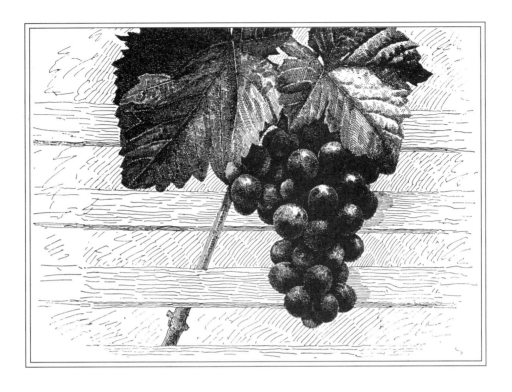

# FRUITS

# A NOTE ON AEROBIC EXERCISE

Exercise physiologists now point out that many forms of exercise, while important to toning and exercising muscle, do little to condition the heart. Many physicians now recommend that healthy adults and children engage in a regular pattern of heart-strengthening activities known as aerobic exercise.

**Aerobic exercise** involves steady uninterrupted activity — at least 12 minutes worth, three or more times a week. During aerobic exercise it's important to work hard enough to increase your heart rate to approximately 75-80 percent of the maximum rate. To find your maximum heart rate, subtract your age from 220. At age 50 your maximum rate would be 170; 80% — 136; 60% — 102.

**Bicycling** works most of the leg muscles. The leg action is more vigorous in bicycling so you can rev up your heart rate and get faster aerobic results. It also is considerably easier on the body than running. Bicycle riding, at a leisurely pace, for 30 minutes, 3 times a week expends 408 calories.

**Jumping rope** is less jarring to the body than running. The force of impact is distributed between both feet, lessening chance of injury. 60-80 skips per minute, for 15 minutes, expends 144 calories.

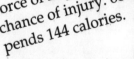

# FRUIT

Discover the many varieties of fruits available, their versatility, and nutritional value. Fruits are refreshing, sweet or tart, juicy, and delicious. They range from the familiar apples, bananas, and oranges to the unfamiliar cherimoya, lychee, and prickly pear.

Virtually all fruits are nutritious — some moderately, some extremely. They provide fiber, minerals, vitamins, carbohydrates, and some protein, with only traces of fat, and NO cholesterol. Which makes fruit not only delicious and easy to eat but GOOD for your health.

As consumers, many of us tend to skip the fruit section of the market, viewing fruit as an unnecessary "extra," and I often hear from friends that fruit is too expensive and just goes to waste anyway. Yet processed and packaged fruit products will be bought instead, with little nutrients, fiber or taste, and at greater expense. Make yourself get into the habit of eating fresh fruit daily, for enjoyment and health benefits. The American Institute for Cancer Research believes that eating fresh fruits daily may help prevent cancer. One way to remind yourself and your family to eat fresh fruit for a snack, lunch, or breakfast is to keep a bowl of fresh fruit as a center piece on the kitchen counter. It makes for a beautiful decoration and reminds you of its availability. Fruit is also great in fresh juices, salads, desserts, and jams.

To help bring fruits back into your diet, or add some variety to your favorite fruits, I have listed a large variety of fruits and their nutritional value. This list should help familiarize you with the new varieties appearing in the fruit sections of the supermarket, and refresh you on the values of the old familiar apple, orange, and pear.

# APPLES

Apples are the most versatile fruit. There are more than 7,000 varieties of apples worldwide, although only 20 varieties make up three quarters of the crop in the United States. Apples have an unbeatable flavor and lots of nutritional value. They provide vitamins A and C, potassium, calcium, carbohydrate, protein, and iron, and are an excellent source of pectin, fiber, magnesium, and B complex. Apples are 85% water. Peak season August through October, but available year round.Some of the more common varieties are:

**Red Delicious** — Deep red in color (sometimes with a slight stripe). The flesh is white, juicy, and mildly sweet. Great in lunches, as a snack, or in salads.

**Golden Delicious** — Whitish green to yellow in color, with a tender skin. Flesh will stay white after cutting, and has a mellow, sweet flavor. Hold their shape well when baked. Golden Delicious are all-purpose apples.

**Winesap** — Usually dark red, and uniformly round. Flesh is very crisp, juicy, and firm. Flavor is a bit tart. An all-purpose apple, good for baking, juicing, drying, or just snacking.

**Rome Beauty** — Bright red, with a spherical shape. Flesh is juicy and aromatic. Best apples for cooking (especially for baked apples).

**Granny Smith** — Rich green skin and a creamy white flesh. A very juicy apple with a tart, pleasant flavor. Great for eating or cooking.

*Purchase* — Look for apples with bright red color (unless they are a "green" variety), and firm to touch. Avoid apples that are excessively bruised, wormy, or brown around the stem end.

*Store* — Keep in refrigerator; will keep 2 weeks or longer. Dried apples should be kept in a closed container in a cool, dry place. Will keep about a year.

*Use* — Delicious raw as a snack, juiced, dried (drying eliminates the vitamin A), excellent baked, stewed, in pies or strudels. Three medium-sized apples will weigh about 3 pounds. One pound cored and sliced apples equals about 4 cups. One apple (medium) has only 80 calories.

## APRICOTS

Apricots are fleshy, one-seeded fruits, close relatives of the almond, peach, cherry, and plum. Ripe apricots are yellow or orange, round, and about 1¹/₂-2 inches in diameter, with sweet flesh. Apricots are 85% water, and provide carbohydrate, calcium, magnesium, and phosphorus. They are high in vitamin A and potassium, with a fair amount of vitamin C, traces of amino acids and other minerals and vitamins. Peak season is June through August, but imported apricots are available December through January. The leading apricot producers are Turkey, Spain, and United States. The U.S. crop comes from California, Washington, and Utah.

*Purchase* — Avoid dull looking or mushy, overripe fruit, or very firm, yellowish-green underripe fruit. Choose plump fruit with a uniform golden-orange color.

*Store* — Will keep about a week in refrigerator.

*Use* — Wash, halve, and remove pit. Apricots are excellent eaten fresh, or in fruit salads, canned, in baked goods, puddings, jams, and sauces.

## AVOCADO

A fruit that is generally used as a vegetable. See avocado in vegetable section, page 75.

## BANANAS

Bananas grow in bunches weighing 60-100 pounds. Each bunch comprises 9-16 clusters called "hands," each containing 12-20 separate bananas (or fingers). Bananas are the world's leading fruit choice. They provide carbohydrates, and are an excellent source of potassium, magnesium, and a considerable amount of vitamin A. They also contain twice as much vitamin C as apples, with folacin, traces of amino acids, minerals, and other vitamins. Bananas are low in fat and protein. Available year round.

*Purchase* — Bananas are at their best when peel is solid yellow, speckled with brown, and firm to the touch. There should be no bruises. Green tips or practically no yellow color means bananas have not yet developed to their full flavor potential.

*Store* — Bananas will continue to ripen at room temperature, and may then be refrigerated. They will keep for 3-5 days (but skin may turn black).

*Use* — Green bananas can be baked or broiled. Uses for bananas are truly endless: Snacking, baking, puddings, sliced on cereals, to mention just a few.

## BERRIES

**Blackberry** — These are hard to find fresh at the markets. You may have to pick them yourself. About 98% of the blackberry crop is processed, frozen, canned, or made into juices or jams. Blackberries provide carbohydrate, fiber, calcium, potassium, magnesium, phosphorus, and vitamins A, C, and B. Peak season is July through September. Store in refrigerator.

**Blueberry** — You will find my favorite berries almost anywhere you look in Alaska. Choose plump, fresh, clean, dry berries, free from insects. Ripeness is indicated by color, which may be black, blue, bluish-black, or purple. Will keep 2-3 days in refrigerator. They provide protein, carbohydrate, fiber, calcium, and vitamins A and C, with traces of amino acids and other vitamins and minerals.

**Boysenberry** — Boysenberries have a purplish-black color, and are larger than blackberries. They are about 95% water, and are a good source of fiber and iron. Boysenberries also provide vitamins A and C, carbohydrate, calcium, and potassium, with traces of other vitamins and minerals.

**Cloud Berry** — A species of raspberry that grows in swampy areas.

**Dewberry** — A type of blackberry; drupes of berries are soft and not closely joined as in other blackberries. Dewberry is grown in the eastern United States.

**Elderberry** — The most common American berry, far higher in vitamin C than citrus fruits. Also provides carbohydrates, fiber, and calcium, is an excellent source of potassium, and a fair source of

**304**

vitamin A, with traces of amino acids, vitamins, and minerals. Flavor is both tart and sweet. Serve fresh; also makes a great wine.

**Gooseberry** — Gooseberries are closely related to currants, except that they are larger and grow singly rather than in clusters. Gooseberries can be white, yellow, or red, as well as green. Rinse and pick them over before using. Great as a snack, in jams, sauces, or stewed. Gooseberries can be substituted for currants or cherries.

**Huckleberry** (Whortleberry) — Resembles a blueberry, but is smaller.

**Loganberry** — This berry is excellent for cooking.

**Mulberry** — Berries are black or white, and have a pleasant flavor. They provide vitamin C, potassium, calcium, carbohydrate, and vitamin A. Tasty eaten fresh, or made into syrup, jam, juice, or wine.

**Oheloberry** — Provides potassium, carbohydrate, vitamins A and C.

**Raspberry** — Raspberries can be red, purple, black, even amber. Peak season is June through August. Raspberries are high in fiber, and provide potassium, vitamins A and C, calcium, carbohydrates, and traces of vitamins and minerals. Avoid berries that are stuck together, wet, or soft. Look for a dry basket without stains on the bottom. Refrigerate unwashed to prevent spoilage. Remember that these berries freeze well. Best eaten raw, alone or with other fresh fruits. 1 cup = 60 calories = 9.1 grams dietary fiber. Also used in pies, tarts, puddings, jams, even stuffings, and vinegars.

**Strawberry** — Strawberries are an excellent source of vitamin C, and also provide fiber, potassium, vitamins A and B, folacin, carbohydrate, traces of amino acids, vitamins, and minerals. Peak season is June through July. Delicious alone, stuffed, dipped in melted chocolate, in tarts, salads, pies, jams — the list goes on and on. Rinse berries before hulling, as water inside the berry can spoil its flavor. Note that most of the vitamin properties are lost in cooking, so while jams are delicious they have only a fraction of the natural vitamins.

## CARAMBOLA (Star Fruit)

The star fruit is an oval-shaped tree melon, 3-8 inches long, with 5 ridges running its length. Has a waxy, shiny appearance. Cut crosswise, it will yield star-shaped slices, which are quite pretty floating in punch. Color may be yellow, greenish, or orange, depending on degree of ripeness and variety. Star fruit has a flavor similar to that of gooseberries, and provides vitamins A and C, with carbohydrate, calcium, potassium, phosphorus, and traces of other vitamins and minerals. It is 91% water and can be quite sour when green. Usually available during our Christmas season. Great in fruit salads and garnishes, or used in baking whenever pineapple is called for. Try with stir-fry chicken, or in a chutney.

## CHERIMOYA

The cherimoya is a member of the anona family. It looks like a large green pine cone, and average size is about the size of a pear, although it can weigh up to a few pounds. It contains tender, light colored, somewhat granular pulp, with a delicate, sweet taste, and a few large, glossy, dark colored non-edible seeds. The cherimoya provides carbohydrate, protein, calcium, phosphorus, and traces of vitamins. It is a poor source of vitamins A and C. Can usually be found in the local Asian market. Handle with care — the skin is easily broken. Eat raw as a fruit, or use as you would bananas. You can also sieve the pulp and use in a variety of drinks or recipes. Cherimoya is native to South and Central America. It is often grown in California and therefore easily accessible.

## CHERRIES

Cherries are small, round, soft fruits, related to peaches and plums. There are two main varieties, sweet and sour. Cherries provide carbohydrate, calcium, potassium, and vitamin C, and are high in vitamin A, with traces of other vitamins and minerals. The sweet cherries are divided into "tender" and "hard" depending on the consistency of the flesh. "Tender" cherries are regular size, with deep pink to red skin and tender juicy flesh, attached to pit. "Hard" cherries are heart-shaped and large with yellowish or dark red skin and firm flesh. The sour cherries are mostly round in shape, usually dark red with juicy, sour flesh. Less common types are:

**Chokecherries** — Small, red, and very tart. They make great syrup.

**Ground Cherries** — Related to tomatoes; round, yellow or green, marble-sized.

*Purchase* — Look for plump, full colored, sweet cherries. Avoid mushy, bruised, shriveled, or dull-skinned cherries. Cherries with dry, brittle stems are overripe. Sour cherries ripen too fast to be marketed fresh, so are only available processed (usually canned).

*Store* — Refrigerate; use within a week or so.

*Use* — Eat fresh as a snack, or in fruit salads, pies, baked goods, and dried. Wash, but do not soak in water. Cherries freeze well.

## COCONUT

Coconut is one of the few fruits that store fats. One-half cup grated coconut contains 142 calories and 12.7 grams of saturated fat (80% fat). Beware of foods that contain coconut oil! Check food labels on crackers, cookies, and most processed and frozen foods. The coconut milk (water) is okay to drink. One cup has only $1/2$ gram fat, and is 95% water, with vitamin C, magnesium, and potassium.

## CRANBERRIES

Cranberries are cousins to blueberries, but are red or pink skinned and larger. Cranberries are a good source of fiber and carbohydrate, and contain vitamins A and C, a fair amount of potassium, with traces of other vitamins and minerals. They are 87% water.

*Purchase* — Choose firm, dry, dark berries. Shriveling and softness indicate poor quality.

*Store* — Will keep several months in refrigerator. They freeze well, and will keep for more than a year frozen.

*Use* — Great, of course, with turkey, pork, or chicken, but also in sauces, jams, pies, and juice.

Note: Sweeten cranberries once they are tender (or skin has split). Cranberries that are sweetened before they are tender develop tough skins.

## CURRANTS *(Black, red, and white)*

Currants are closely related to gooseberries, but are smaller and grow in clusters. Currants have a delicious tart flavor. They provide calcium, iron, carbohydrate, fiber, magnesium, and phosphorus, and are an excellent source of potassium, with vitamins A and C, and traces of other vitamins and minerals. Fresh currants are not often available in the markets. Red and white currants are considered to be lower in potassium and vitamin C than the black ones. Dried currants contain no vitamin C, but are rich in potassium, fiber, calcium, and iron. They are like miniature raisins, and are great in pies, jams, and sauces, or as a snack. Zante currants are small raisins that resemble dried currants.

## DATES

The nutritional value of dates is their high sugar content: 60% in soft dates, and as much as 70% in the dry types. They provide some protein, carbohydrate, fiber, ash, calcium, iron, and vitamin A, with traces of other vitamins and minerals. They are also high in potassium, although they contain little or no vitamin C.

*Purchase* — Look for plump dates with good color and smooth, glossy skin. If they are shriveled and dull, they have been stored too long. When purchasing dried dates, look for well-shaped, whole dates. Avoid broken or moldy ones. Packaged dried dates often have corn syrup added to keep them moist.

*Store* — Keep fresh dates refrigerated in airtight containers to prevent absorption of other food odors. Soft dates are best stored in a cool, dry place; use within 6 months. Dates freeze well.

*Use* — Serve fresh, alone, puréed in a milk shake, or in a variety of recipes: Stuffed, stewed, in cookies, fruit cakes, puddings, with chicken, or in breads.

## FIGS

They belong to the family Moraceae (along with mulberries and breadfruit). Figs are loaded with natural food energy (they are 55% calories). They provide carbohydrate, are high in calcium and iron, and are a good source of potassium. Fresh figs also contain vitamin A, with traces of amino acids and other vitamins and minerals. They are 79% water, contain no sodium, and are high in fiber. Dried figs are 266 calories per 100 grams, fresh or canned figs are 65-80 calories per 100 grams (about $3^1/_2$ ounces). Color (green, white, red or purple) is not a sign of ripeness — softness is. Peak season is June through November. Fresh figs are highly perishable; eat right away or store in the refrigerator. Do not peel; simply rinse and remove stalk. Choose unbruised fruit. Keep dried figs in a cool, dry place. Eat as a snack, in jams, stewed, stuffed, added to baked goods, or even pickled. If the surface develops sugar, dip into lukewarm water. Figs can be substituted for apricots in recipes.

## GRAPEFRUIT

Grapefruits are thought to have developed from the pomelo (see page 320), or as a hybrid between an orange and a pomelo. They provide vitamins A and C, carbohydrate, calcium, potassium, and traces of other vitamins and minerals. White and pink varieties are grown. White grapefruits are usually small and quite tart. Pink grapefruits are large, with a sweet-tart flavor, or small and thin-skinned. All have yellow skins that can be smooth or rough. Some varieties are seedless. Good quality grapefruits are firm and springy to the touch. Avoid grapefruits with soft, wilted, or moldy spots. For breakfast just cut in half and serve, or drizzle with honey and broil for a couple of minutes. Grapefruit juice is a breakfast favorite, but try it in place of lemon juice in salads, or with chicken and lamb.

## GRAPES

Grapes provide the richest fruit source of chromium and are a good source of potassium. They provide carbohydrate, calcium, vitamins A, B-complex, and C, small amounts of protein and fat, with traces of amino acids, and other vitamins and minerals.

**Concord Grapes** — Flavorful, dark purple, used as table grapes, or in wines, jams, and jellies.

**Thompson Grapes** — Seedless, light green, medium to large in size. Thompson grapes comprise 95% of all raisins produced.

**Ribier Grapes** — Large purple-black, mildly sweet, available July through February.

**Emperor Grapes** — Large red grapes, with a cherry-like flavor. Available September through March.

*Purchase* — Grapes do not ripen after harvesting. When purchasing, choose brightly-colored grapes attached to green, pliable stems. Grapes should be wrinkle-free and firm. Avoid leaking grapes.

*Store* — Grapes will stay fresh for several days in the refrigerator.

*Use* — Wash and serve grapes alone, or in a variety of recipes. There are endless ways to use them: In chicken and seafood dishes, salads, desserts, garnishes, and of course, dried. Raisins are a great take-along snack for children.

## GUAVA

Guavas are an excellent source of vitamins A and C, and a good source of potassium and fiber, with carbohydrate and traces of amino acids, vitamins, and minerals.

**Common Guava** — Yellow to green when ripe, and very sweet.

**Strawberry Guava** — Reddish purple on the outside and white on the inside. Tastes like a strawberry.

**Pineappe Guava** — Usually green-tinted with red, with a pleasant aroma and mixed pineapple/strawberry flavor. Commonly round or pear shaped, 1-4 inches in diameter. Contains many small seeds with an unusual, gritty texture. Choose firm, unblemished guavas. Peel and eat raw, seeds and all, alone or in fruit salads, or cooked in pies or jams.

## JUJUBE (Chinese date)

The jujube is rust in color, and must be left to slightly wither after picking so the pulp becomes spongy and sweet. It provides a good source of potassium and vitamin C, with fiber, carbohydrate, and traces of other vitamins and minerals. The jujube is sold fresh, dried, canned or in juice. Eat raw or use in baking; it is said to be very soothing to sore throats.

## KIWI

Kiwis (or Chinese gooseberries) are plum-sized, with a dull brown, fuzzy skin. Inside, the kiwi has brilliant green pulp, white in the center, with many very small black seeds. Kiwis are rich in vitamin C, and provide carbohydrate, vitamin A, potassium, and calcium, with traces of other vitamins and minerals. The kiwi flavor is a blend of tropical tartness and sweetness. Choose ripe kiwis that yield to gentle pressure. Firm kiwis can be ripened at room temperature. Cut in half and eat with a spoon right out of the shell, or peel and slice. Use as a snack, in salads, desserts, tarts, garnishes, and jams.

## KUMQUATS

Kumquats are closely related to citrus fruits, but are only $1^1/_2$-2 inches in diameter. They are juicy and sweet with a crisp tartness, few seeds, and an edible rind. Kumquats are high in fiber, and a good source of potassium; they provide calcium, magnesium, phosphorus, and vitamins A and C. Choose healthy looking kumquats, without bruises, wrinkles, or soft spots. They should be heavy for their size.

## LEMONS

Lemons are a good source of vitamin C, with potassium, carbohydrate, vitamin A, folacin, and traces of other vitamins and minerals. Most of us know that lemons are for making lemonade, but we overlook their many other uses. Lemon juice is an excellent salt substitute, meat tenderizer, or added seasoning. Uses for lemons are endless, and since they can be kept in the refrigerator for up to a month, there is no reason to be without a fresh squeeze of lemon juice. Choose the largest and freshest looking. Avoid lemons with soft spots, or those that are dry and wrinkled. Be very sure to wash lemons well before using the rind. In some cases the lemons have been treated with sprays, dyes, or wax. This is true for any fruit rind to be used.

## LIMES

Limes and lemons are major fruit crops: 5 million metric tons are produced annually worldwide. Limes look like green lemons. They provide moderate amounts of vitamin C, potassium, calcium, and carbohydrate, with traces of vitamins and minerals. Choose firm, blemish-free limes; avoid any that are dry or wrinkled. Use same as lemons in a variety of ways — stir-fry, salads, seafood, sauces, chicken, desserts, garnish.

## LOQUAT  (Japanese Medlar)

Loquats are an excellent source of potassium, and provide carbohydrate, calcium, and vitamin A, with traces of other vitamins and minerals. Their sizes vary from gooseberry size to 5 centimeters long and 4 centimeters wide. Loquats have thin, waxy, yellow or golden skin, and large black stones. The pulp is juicy with a crunchy texture, and the flavor is both sweet and acid. Outer skin is edible. If cooking loquats, do not peel until after they are cooked. Fresh lemon juice helps bring out the flavor.

## LYCHEE (Litchi)

Lychees are 82% water and provide vitamin C, potassium, carbohydrate, and traces of other vitamins and minerals. Ripe lychees are about the size of plums, with very thin, deep pink/red skin that easily separates from the fruit. Inside is a fleshy juicy white pulp covering a large black seed. Lychees are best chilled and eaten fresh.

They are available dried or canned, and are sometimes used to sweeten meat and poultry dishes. Will keep up to 3 months in refrigerator; they also freeze well. Found in most Asian markets.

## MANGO

The mango belongs to the same family as cashew and pistachio nuts, and comes in many varieties and shapes. It has juicy orange flesh and skin that is either yellow, reddish-orange, green, or rainbow in color. It is an excellent source of vitamin A, with potassium, carbohydrate, vitamin C, and traces of other vitamins and minerals. Its flavor is distinctive, both sweet and sour. Choose a ripe mango that yields slightly to pressure. Avoid mangos with black spotted skin — this indicates overripe fruit. Underripe fruit will ripen at room temperature. Ripe fruit will keep for a couple of days in the refrigerator. Best eaten raw, or peeled and cut up in a salad, in chutney, pies, jams, ice cream, or with seafood.

## MELONS

Melons are the favorite fruit of many. A ripe, juicy, sweet slice of melon is both irresistible and refreshing. Melons come in many shapes and colors, and are related to cucumbers and squash. Melons provide potassium, vitamin A, carbohydrate, amino acids, and traces of other vitamins and minerals. Choose melons that seem heavy for their size, free of mold or soft spots. Keep melon wrapped well when chilling in the refrigerator, or its smell may permeate other foods. The melon seeds are edible. Rinse, pat dry, and roast seeds in a slow oven until lightly toasted.

The most common types of melon are listed below. Try them all — you will enjoy them.

**Canary** — These melons have a rounded-oblong shape, and when ripe the rind turns from light yellow to intense yellow. The flesh is firm, and ranges from light green to white in color.

**Cantaloupe** — Choose plump, oval-shaped melon, with greenish skin and a coarse white netting. Cantaloupe should yield slightly at the stem end when pressed. Cantaloupe is 90% water, high in vitamin A (in beta-carotene form), vitamin C, folacin, potassium, calcium, magnesium, carbohydrate, fiber, and traces of other vitamins and minerals. Has a juicy, sweet flavor and orange flesh.

**Casaba** — Casaba is a round melon with a pointed end, and a ridged and furrowed rind. The rind turns a rich yellow at maturity. Has a pleasant aroma, with juicy, sweet flesh. Provides vitamin C, potassium, and carbohydrate, with traces of minerals.

**Crenshaw** — Globe-shaped and pointed at stem end with a shallow furrow, the Crenshaw is a cross between Persian and Casaba melons. When melon is ripe, the rind is medium to bright yellow, and stem end should yield slightly to pressure. Flesh is an orange/pink color, very perishable, and bruises easily.

**Honeydew** — Green honeydew melon is oval, with a pale green, waxy skin. The rind turns a creamy color when ripe and ready to eat, the blossom end yields slightly when pressed, and the aroma is pronounced. This melon is very juicy and wonderfully sweet. Provides calcium, vitamins A and C, traces of other vitamins and minerals, and is high in potassium.

**Kiwano** (Horned Melon) — This fruit is a member of the melon family, closely related to honeydew or cantaloupe, as well as the cucumber. Horned melons are native to Africa, but are also grown in other areas including the warm parts of the United States. The husk is usually orange, with green pulp and edible seeds. They are oval-shaped, 6 inches or less in length, with numerous soft spines. Will keep 6 months after being picked if stored at room temperature.

**Orange-Fleshed Melon** — These melons are smaller than the green honeydew, with a texture and flavor similar to that of cantaloupe. When ripe, the rind changes in color from almost white to light orange.

**Persian** — Looks like a slightly flattened cantaloupe. The rind is dark green with a fine gray netting. Persian melons have a sweet flavor and dense, orange-pink flesh.

**Watermelon** — Provides potassium, vitamin A, carbohydrate, amino acids, traces of other vitamins and minerals, and is 91% water. Oblong or slightly rounded, watermelons vary greatly in size. The rind can be dark or light green in color, with or without stripes. Choose a melon with a symmetrical shape and a hollow sound when tapped. It is easier to choose a cut watermelon than a whole one. Look for fresh, firm texture, and dark red flesh (which indicates sweetness). Other varieties of watermelon are:

*Calsweet or Triplesweet* — Oblong melons with a striped dark skin.

*Citron* — A variety of watermelon that has a hard thick white flesh. Rind may be candied or pickled.

*Orchid Sweet* — Dark green skin with yellow flesh.

*Picnic or Peacock* — Smaller, rounder melons with dark green skin.

*Santa Claus or Christmas* — Oblong-shaped melon with green-yellow rind, and firm white flesh. Available year round.

*Texas Gray* — Evenly colored light green skin.

Watermelon is great as a snack, or in fruit salads, jams, and pickles.

## NECTARINES

Nectarines are related to apricots and peaches. They are round, with a slight crease or groove from stem to blossom end. They are golden in color with a blush of red, and contain an almond-shaped hard seed. Nectarines provide vitamins A and C, potassium, carbohydrate, and traces of minerals and vitamins. Avoid nectarines that are hard and green, or bruised, moldy, or too soft. Softness indicates a woolly or mealy texture that cannot be changed by cooking. Nectarines usually do not become sweeter after picking, so eat as fresh as possible. Handle with care to prevent bruising — they are highly perishable.

## ORANGES

Oranges are the most popular fruits in the United States, and are available year round. The 4 main types are Navel, Valencia, Seville, and Blood oranges.

All oranges are an excellent source of vitamin C, and a good source of potassium, carbohydrate, calcium, folacin, and vitamin A, with traces of amino acids, minerals, and vitamins. Choose oranges that are unbruised, unwrinkled, feel heavy for their size, and have a soft shine to the skin. Peel and serve sections alone, or with other fruits, in salads or jams; use for fresh juice, or in a variety of recipes. Sweet oranges have a weak flavor when cooked and are best eaten raw. Oranges freeze well. If you want the most juice from an orange, some suggest warming it. A quick way to do this is to pour boiling water over the orange and let sit a few minutes (3-5). Another hint — if you wish to have perfect segments of an orange, peel it and chill till very firm but not frozen. This makes it easier to cut down between the segment skins and remove perfectly shaped pieces.

**Navels** — Usually large, seedless, and sweet. Skin is thick and bumpy. Navels are great as a snack.

**Seville** — These oranges are important in cooking. They have a rough, dark orange skin, and lots of seeds. Sevilles are very aromatic but have a sour flavor. Great in marmalade, liqueurs, or candied.

**Valencias** — Sizes vary from small to grapefruit size. Skin is thin and smooth. They are sweet and juicy, with many seeds.

**Blood Oranges** — Sweet and juicy, with thin skins that are hard to peel. Named for the often red juice these oranges contain.

## LOOSE-SKINNED ORANGES:

These include Mandarins, Tangerines, and Satsumas. Loose-skinned oranges are more perishable than the tight-skinned varieties. They provide vitamin A, potassium, a small amount of vitamin C, and traces of amino acids, vitamins, and minerals.

**Mandarin** — Chinese in origin, mandarin skins are orange-red, and separate from the flesh easily. Slightly tart flavor with lots of seeds.

**Tangerines** — African in origin, there are several varieties, often mistakenly called Mandarins.

*Kinnow* — Thin-skinned, yellow, hard to peel.

*Clementines* — Larger than the other loose-skinned oranges. Has an orange, bumpy skin. Slightly tart but juicy.

*Temple* — Tangerine and orange cross. Fairly large, with a tangy flavor, excellent for snacking.

*Tangelos* — Tangerine and grapefruit cross. Tangelos taste similar to tangerines; they are not much like the grapefruit side of their family in either flavor or appearance. Slightly tart and juicy with lots of seeds.

**Satsumas** — Japanese in origin. They are very small, sweet, and almost seedless.

## PAPAYA *(Pawpaw, Papa, or Papaw)*

A large pear-shaped fruit, with a smooth skin that turns from green to yellow when ripe. Ripest papaya is nearly all yellow or orange. Some grow to 18 inches long, but the most common are about 6 inches long. The pulp is soft and yellow orange in color, the flavor and texture is similar to the melons. Papayas are high in vitamin A, and provide calcium, fiber, carbohydrate, potassium, traces of amino acids, vitamins, and minerals, and are 89% water. You cannot go wrong with a papaya. One papaya is equivalent to 3 oranges worth of vitamin C. It has an enzyme — papain — that breaks down protein, which aids digestion, and it makes a great meat tenderizer. The flesh is similar to a mushy melon, although sometimes it has a peppery taste. The flavor is heightened with a little fresh lemon. Cut the papaya in half lengthwise, and remove and discard the black peppercorn-size seeds. Eat a papaya as you would a melon. Refreshing for breakfast with a sprinkle of lime juice, or in a fruit drink, salads, jams, even baked. Papayas can be substituted for melons in most recipes. They keep their flavor when cooked.

## PASSION FRUIT *(Granadilla)*

The passion fruit is 73% water and provides vitamin A, niacin, potassium, carbohydrate, traces of other minerals, and is high in fiber. The fruit is egg shaped with a wrinkled, leathery skin that may appear overripe. Passion fruit has a punchy sweet flavor, with a wonderful fragrance. It has numerous crunchy, edible seeds, or you can sieve the seeds out and use the pulp. Since passion fruits are usually individually priced, choose the largest you can.

## PEACHES

Peaches are a good source of potassium and an excellent source of vitamin A, with carbohydrate, amino acids, and traces of vitamins and minerals. Avoid peaches that are soft or bruised. Softness indicates a mealy texture, which cannot be changed even with cooking. Wash, peel, and eat alone, or use in numerous recipes — pies, sherbets, stewed, stuffed, baked or in jam.

## PEARS

Winter meals can be given new life with the addition of fresh pears. As appetizers, pears go well with many cheeses, especially gouda, Swiss, and brie. Pears are also wonderful in salads and desserts, and can even be used as a garnish. Like citrus fruits, pears are a source of vitamins A and C, potassium, iron, magnesium, and phosphorus, and offer considerable amounts of easily digested fiber. Fresh pears are 80% water.

Popular varieties:

**Anjou** — May be light green or yellow-green, but color is no clue to ripeness. Pressure testing is the only way to determine the ripeness of the fruit. When it yields to gentle pressure at the stem end, it is ready to eat. The Anjou has creamy flesh with a sweet, slightly spicy flavor. Excellent by itself, in salads, or with cheeses.

**Bartlett** — Bell-shaped pear, turns from green to yellow as it ripens, and sometimes has a crimson blush on yellow skin. Flesh is white, smooth, and juicy — perfect for snacking, salads, and desserts. Bartlett pears are also good for canning. Available from July through December.

**Bosc** — When ripe, the Bosc pear has a golden-brown skin, with russeting over golden-yellow. Gentle pressure at the stem end indicates when it is ready to eat. Delicious eaten fresh, but also excellent for baking, poaching, and cooking because it holds its shape and flavor well. Available in September, with increasing availability throughout the winter, and usually available until June.

**Comice** — Turns from green to greenish-yellow when ripe, and frequently has a crimson blush. Comice is an extremely juicy pear of high quality, with smooth flesh and sweet flavor. At its best during the holiday season, and favored in fruit baskets. Available from October through March.

**Nelis** — Medium to small pear, with almost no neck definition. Its skin is light brown russeting over light green, and becomes more golden when ripe. The Nelis pear has sweet, creamy flesh and good cooking qualities. Since pears are small, they make great snacks. Available October through April.

**Red Bartlett** — The same as Bartlett pears, but the skin is entirely red. Available August through October.

## PERSIMMONS (Kaki)

Persimmons are considered to be one of the best-known fruits of the Orient. Plum-shaped or round, 2-4 inches in diameter, they resemble tomatoes in many ways. Persimmons are high in vitamin A, and provide carbohydrate, calcium, potassium, and traces of other vitamins and minerals, also providing a high percentage of protein. They have a pleasant, spicy-sweet flavor when fully ripe. Beware of unripe persimmons — the fruit has a pungent flavor if not fully ripened. Choose fruit that is soft but not mushy. The fruit that appears a bit too ripe and slightly wrinkled is just right. Persimmons are delicious plain, or with a bit of cinnamon, nutmeg, ginger, or all 3, or use a sprinkle of fresh lemon juice. Use in salads, cakes, puddings, or breads; they can be candied or even puréed into popsicles. Always check to see where the persimmons were grown. If they are labeled Sharon (persimmons from the Sharon Valley in Israel) they can be eaten right away, firm or soft. You can eat skin, seeds, and all.

## PINEAPPLE

The pineapple is a fair source of vitamin A, with potassium, vitamin C, and traces of vitamins, minerals, and amino acids. Choose fragrant, unbruised pineapple with a tinge of gold or red, and fresh green leaves. Remove core and shell, slice into rings or chunks and serve. Add to a variety of recipes from yogurt to cake or use in salads, stir-fry, chicken dishes, jam, etc. If using in gelatin, you must substitute canned or cooked pineapple — fresh pineapple does not allow gelatin to jell. Pineapple does not freeze well.

## PLANTAINS

Yellow plantains actually range in color from green to yellow to red, and to black when fully ripe. Plantains have a higher starch content than bananas, which makes it necessary to cook them before eating. They are high in vitamin A, with amino acids, potassium, vitamin C, and carbohydrate, and traces of other minerals and vitamins. Can be stored in refrigerator for about 3 days after ripe. Peel and sauté or roast in skins. Used more as a vegetable than a fruit.

## PLUMS

Plums are a good source of potassium, and provide amino acids, vitamin A, carbohydrate, and traces of vitamins and minerals. Avoid bruised plums, or plums with damaged skins. Tough skins may be peeled.

**Damson Plum** — Certain varieties of damson plums are used to make dried prunes.

## POMEGRANATE

Deep red on the outside, about the size of an apple. Outer skin is thick and leathery. Look for large fruit with unbroken skin that feels heavy for its size. Pomegranate is a good source of potassium and carbohydrate, with traces of vitamins and minerals. Poor source of vitamin C. Flavor is sweet and acidic. Serve as a snack (it's a great take-along snack), or in salads, marinades, and as a garnish. The pomegranate juice is called grenadine. Cut the skin with a sharp knife and peel back, or cut in half and spoon out seeds. Pomegranates are fun to eat because of all the seeds.

## POMELO

Pomelo is a large fruit, usually 5-10 inches in diameter, with a very thick, yellow rind. Its appearance and flavor resemble a grapefruit. Pomelo provides vitamin C, potassium, carbohydrate, and traces of vitamins and minerals. Remove the rind and tough membrane around each section. The flesh breaks into sections. Eat alone, or in salads.

## *PRICKLY PEAR FRUIT (Opuntia or Indian Fig)*

Not related to pears, this thorny, elongated, apple-shaped fruit is actually a type of cactus. Flesh is sweet but seedy. The skin turns from green to yellow and red.

## *PRICKLY PEAR PAD (Indian Fig)*

Has spiny pads, can be found in the fresh fruit section of the market. Provides potassium, magnesium, calcium, vitamin C, carbohydrates, and traces of other vitamins. The seeds run through the flesh and they are pleasant and add to the texture. Prickly pears have a sweet flavor. Wash pads, carefully cut away all the spines, then peel the skin from pad. Slice crosswise into a long section. Eat raw, sprinkled with fresh lime or lemon juice, or steamed or boil until tender.

## *PRUNES*

Prunes are dried plums. They are an excellent source of vitamin A, calcium, potassium, and iron. Prunes are also high in fiber: Four prunes have 5.4 grams of fiber, and are 32% water. Will keep for months in a cool dry place, refrigeration not needed. Avoid damaged or bruised prunes.

## *QUINCE*

The quince is shaped like both apples and pears. When ripe, fruit is hard, lemon yellow, and aromatic. Flavor is tart when eaten raw; some prefer a sweetener. Quince is a good source of fiber and vitamin C, and provides potassium, vitamin A, carbohydrate, and traces of other minerals and vitamins. Pare and core before cooking, and add to stews, jams, pies, chutneys, or puddings. Quince are seldom available at the market, so choose whatever you can get.

## RHUBARB

Rhubarb has sleek green and red stalks, with wide curly leaves. The leaves and the roots are TOXIC, containing high levels of oxalic acid. Stalks are edible, with a tart-sour flavor. Rhubarb provides potassium, vitamin A, calcium, carbohydrate, and traces of other minerals and vitamins. Choose young pink stems for best flavor; thick rhubarb becomes coarse and stringy. Use in wines, pies, tarts, jams, desserts, and sauces. Rhubarb can be frozen before or after cooking.

## ROSEHIPS

Rosehips, the red seed pod of the wild or garden rose, are one of the best natural sources of vitamin C. Tests show it to be far superior to the vitamin C in orange juice, with the northern U.S. variety being richer than that grown in the south. Three rosehips equal 1 orange.

**Raw rosehips** — Grind 2 pounds cleaned rosehips, add 1 pint water and bring to a boil. Let boil 20 minutes covered. Rub through a sieve, pour into small jars, seal, and process in a hot water bath for 20 minutes. This purée makes a nice addition to soups, puddings, and stocks. Add just before serving (1 part purée to 3 parts stock).

**Dried rosehips** — Cut rosehips in half and remove seeds. Dry in a slow oven. Great added to granola or cereals, cooked with fruit, or pulverized and added to baked products — and of course, that welcome cup of hot tea.

## SAPODILLA

A soft brown fruit about the size of a kiwi, it has sweet brown flesh with black seeds. Provides carbohydrate, and is a good source of potassium, vitamin C, traces of amino acids, vitamins, and minerals. Serve the fresh fruit raw with fresh lime juice, or mix into fruit salads, puddings, or creams.

## SOURSOP *(Custard Apple)*

Fruit is green with rows of spines, and typically weighs up to 6 pounds. Soursops are a good source of fiber, and also provide potassium, calcium, traces of amino acids, vitamins, and minerals. Serve raw with a bit of sweetener, or in salads or jams.

## WATERMELONS

See melons, pages 313-315.

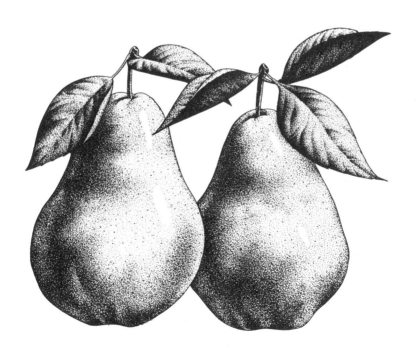

## FRUIT SALAD
## WITH STRAWBERRY YOGURT  3-4 servings

*2 kiwi fruit — peeled and sliced*
*½ cup cantaloupe — cut into bite-sized pieces*
*½ cup watermelon — cut into bite-sized pieces (remove seeds)*
*½ cup pineapple — cut into bite-sized pieces (fresh or canned)*
*1 cup strawberries — cleaned and quartered*
*1 cup grapes (seedless) — washed and drained*
*1½ cups lowfat strawberry yogurt*

Combine all fruit, fold in strawberry yogurt. Chill before serving.

## POPPY SEED FRUIT SALAD
## (BUG SALAD)  4 servings

*1 banana — sliced*
*1 red apple — cut into bite-sized pieces (leave skin on)*
*1 small cantaloupe — cubed*
*1 orange — cut each segment in 3*
*2 Tablespoons lemon juice*
*¾ cup pecan halves — do not chop*
*¼ cup poppy seeds*

Mix all ingredients and chill well before serving. Serve plain or with yogurt.

# STUFFED STRAWBERRIES

*1 pint strawberries — washed*
*1 - 8 ounce package cream cheese — softened*
*½ cup semi-sweet chocolate chips*

Clean strawberries and remove a bit of the core. Stuff each strawberry with softened cream cheese. In a double boiler or ceramic pot, melt chocolate chips over low heat until smooth and creamy. Dip tips of strawberries into creamy chocolate and place berries tips up on serving dish. Serve well chilled.

# FRESH FRUIT SALAD                    4 servings

*2 mangos — peeled and sliced*
*1 pint strawberries — washed and cut in half*
*2 kiwi fruit — peeled and sliced*
*8 prunes — stewed (steamed till plump)*
*⅓ cup whipping cream*
*1 teaspoon vanilla*
*2 heaping Tablespoons plain nonfat yogurt*

Set out 4 serving dishes and divide fruit evenly between them. In a small bowl, whip cream and vanilla until soft peaks form, then fold in yogurt. Place a dab of whipped cream mixture on top of each serving.

## FRUIT SALAD FOR TWO

*2 kiwi fruit — peeled and sliced*
*1 banana — sliced*
*About 5 strawberries — washed and quartered*
*¼ cup whipping cream*
*½ teaspoon vanilla*
*2 Tablespoons fresh coconut — shredded*

Divide fruit between two serving bowls. Partially whip cream. Add vanilla and continue whipping cream until fluffy, then fold in coconut. Place a dab of whipped coconut cream on top of each serving of fruit. Sprinkle with cinnamon and serve.

## FRUIT TOSS SALAD                                     4 servings

*1¼ cups watermelon — remove seeds and cut into 1-inch cubes*
*1½ cups cantaloupe — cut into small pieces or melon balls*
*1½ cups strawberries — washed and quartered*

Toss fruit in bowl and chill.

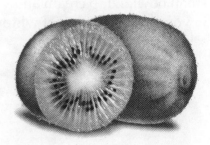

## FRUIT DRINK

Approximately 2 cups

*1 banana*
*1 peach — washed with pit removed, peeled if desired*
*1 cup orange juice*

Combine all ingredients in blender. Blend until smooth. (If desired, add 3-5 ice cubes and blend well.)


## BANANA DRINK

3-4 servings

*2 bananas — peeled and sliced*
*2 cups lowfat or nonfat milk*
*½ cup plain nonfat yogurt*
*½ teaspoon vanilla*
*½ cup orange juice*
*4-6 ice cubes — cracked*

Combine all ingredients in a blender on liquid setting until ice is liquid. Serve immediately.

## CANTALOUPE DRINK

4 servings

1 cup cantaloupe — chopped
½ cup banana — sliced
½ cup orange juice
¼ cup nonfat yogurt
4 ice cubes — cracked

Combine all ingredients in blender on liquid setting until ice is liquid. Serve immediately.

## FRUIT DISH FOR TWO

1 cup apricots — clean, remove pits and chop into bite-sized pieces
1½ cups fresh or canned pineapple — chopped into bite-sized pieces

Combine apricots and pineapple in a salad bowl, chill, and serve. This combination is a refreshing snack.

# PRUNE WHIP

4 servings

*1½ cups prunes — remove pits and chop*
*1½ cups water*
*½ cup raisins*
*¼ teaspoon allspice*
*½ teaspoon cinnamon*
*½ cup plain nonfat yogurt*

In a saucepan, combine prunes, water, and raisins. Simmer, covered, about 10 minutes. Add allspice and cinnamon, and let simmer a few more minutes. Remove from heat and let cool a few minutes. Place prune mixture in blender. Add yogurt and whip until smooth. Makes a great snack, dessert, or even breakfast.

# YOGURT FRENCH TOAST

2-3 servings

*2 eggs*
*¼ cup 2% or nonfat milk*
*¼ teaspoon cinnamon*
*¼ cup plain nonfat yogurt*
*Drop of vanilla*
*Whole wheat bread*
*Dab of margarine*

In a bowl, beat eggs. Add milk, cinnamon, yogurt, and vanilla, and mix well. Coat bread slices in egg mixture on both sides. Fry in a hot skillet with a dab of margarine (or unsalted butter), browning both sides. Serve with syrup, peanut butter, fruit, or favorite jam.

# FRENCH STYLE APPLE PIE

9-inch pie

*1 unbaked 9-inch pie crust (see page 270)*
*6-8 apples — peeled and sliced thin*
*2 Tablespoons molasses*
*1 teaspoon cinnamon*
*2 Tablespoons fresh lemon juice*
*1 cup oats — raw flakes or rolled oats if you prefer*
*½ cup nuts — chopped*
*½ cup unsweetened coconut — optional (coconut is high in fat content)*
*2 Tablespoons margarine — melted*

Preheat oven to 350°

In a large bowl, combine sliced apples, molasses, cinnamon, and fresh lemon juice; toss and set aside. In another bowl, combine oats, nuts, and coconut. Add melted margarine and mix well. Place apples in the lined pie plate. Cover apples with oat mixture. Cover crust edges with strips of foil, and cover top of pie with foil. Bake for 30 minutes, remove top foil and continue to bake 15 minutes longer to brown top. Total cooking time approximately 50 minutes.

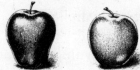

# FRESH BERRY PIE

Select ripe berries — blackberries, blueberries, huckleberries, boysenberries, etc. Berries picked at the height of the season are sweeter and require less sugar than the earlier berries. Very tart berries may need more sugar than recipe calls for. Wash berries, and drain well. Pick the berries over and remove stems and hulls.

Make crust for 9-inch 2-crust pie. Line pie pan with bottom crust. (See page 270.)

*³/₄ cup brown sugar*
*¹/₃ cup unbleached white flour*
*¹/₂ teaspoon cinnamon*
**4 cups fresh berries**
**1 Tablespoon margarine**

Preheat oven to 425°

Mix together sugar, flour, and cinnamon. Add to berries and mix lightly. Turn into pastry-lined pie pan. Dot with margarine, cover with top crust, and seal and flute edges. Cover edges with a thin strip of foil to prevent excess browning. Cut a few slits in top crust to allow steam to escape. Bake about 40 minutes or until crust is nicely browned. Serve slightly warm or cold.

---

### BERRY PICKING

Picking berries in the Alaska forest and picking berries in the city next to the freeway are two extremes but you must be aware of WHERE you are picking your berries in either case. Always stay at least 15 feet from the roadside and check surrounding foliage for withering, curling or twisting that would indicate recent spraying. Do not eat berries at parks because of frequent sprayings of herbicides. Although officials say it is safe because they do not spray once the fruit starts growing, there is not a herbicide label yet that says fruits and vegetables treated with it should be eaten. Any berries that you do pick should be washed with running water before eating or cooking. I soak my berries a few minutes in salted water to remove any worms or insects.

---

# FAST CHEESE PIE

Yields 9-inch pie

**Crust:**
1½ cups crushed whole wheat graham crackers
¼ cup sugar
3 Tablespoons butter — melted

Preheat oven to 375°

Mix ingredients well. Press firmly into a 9-inch pie plate. Bake for 5-6 minutes, or until edges are browned. Remove and cool.

Lower oven to 350°

**Filling:**
1½ pounds cream cheese
4 eggs — discard 2 yolks
½ cup honey
2 Tablespoons fresh lemon juice
1 Tablespoon lemon rind — grated

Whip filling ingredients together, pour into cooled crust. Bake 10-12 minutes, until just firm. Cool.

# BAKED APPLES DELUXE
6 servings

*6 red apples (Romes or Delicious) — medium to large*
*½ cup dried apples — chopped*
*½ cup raisins — chopped*
*½ cup nuts — chopped*
*1 cup orange juice*
*2 Tablespoons bran*
*2 Tablespoons molasses*
*1 Tablespoon orange rind — grated*
*1½ Tablespoons margarine*
*¼ teaspoon fresh nutmeg — grated*
*2 Tablespoons plain nonfat yogurt*
*Extra yogurt for topping — optional*

Preheat oven to 350°

Wash and core apples and place in a baking dish. Mix dried apples, raisins, and nuts together. Fill each cored apple with apple-raisin-nut mixture. In a saucepan, heat orange juice, bran, molasses, orange rind, margarine, nutmeg, and yogurt. Mix well. Pour sauce into center of each apple. Baste sides. Bake for 30-35 minutes. Baste while cooking. To serve, ladle sauce over each apple; put 1 large Tablespoon of plain yogurt on top of each apple (optional), ladle a little more sauce on top, and serve.

Whipped cream or ice cream can be used in place of yogurt as a topping.

## APRICOT JAM WITH SUNFLOWER SEEDS

Yields 6¹/₂ pints

*6 cups apricots — rinsed and chopped (do not peel)*
*1 box powdered pectin (containing no sugar or preservatives)*
*1¹/₂ cups honey (favorite kind)*
*¹/₄ cup lemon juice*
*1 cup unsalted sunflower seeds*

Place apricots in a large kettle. Mash them and heat slowly. Once the juice begins to run, heat may be increased. Cook the apricots for about 15 minutes. Add pectin and mix well. Bring to a boil, add honey, lemon juice, and sunflower seeds, and stir well. Bring to a rolling boil and cook for 5 minutes. Remove from heat. Spoon into hot jars, leaving about a ¹/₂ inch space at the top of jar. Seal, process in a boiling water bath for 10 minutes. (See next page for hot water bath.)

## PAPAYA JAM WITH ALMONDS

Yields 6¹/₂ pints

*6 cups papaya*
*1 box powdered pectin (containing no sugar or preservatives)*
*1¹/₂ cups honey*
*¹/₄ cup fresh lemon juice*
*¹/₂ teaspoon cinnamon*
*¹/₄ teaspoon allspice*
*1 cup almond slivers*

Use same directions as above.

# *APRICOT-PAPAYA JAM*  Yields 6½ pints

*4 cups apricots*
*2 cups papayas*
*1 box powdered pectin (containing no sugar or preservatives)*
*1½ cups honey*
*¼ cup lemon juice*

Use directions for apricot jam with sunflower seeds (previous page).

---

## *HOT WATER BATH*

The Hot Water Bath Method is used to process fruits, tomatoes, and pickles. These are acidic foods and can be safely canned in boiling water.

You can purchase a special hot water bath kettle, but any large metal container can double as a hot water bath kettle if it is deep enough that the water is well over the tops of the jars and has space to boil freely (2-4 inches). The kettle must have a rack to hold jars at least 1 inch above the bottom of the kettle. The rack may be metal or wood, but must allow the water to circulate. The kettle must also have a cover, which helps keep the water at a good rolling boil. Place the jars of food on the rack in the kettle far enough apart to allow the circulation of water around them. Start counting processing time as soon as the water in the kettle resumes a good rolling boil after you have added the jars. Keep the water boiling constantly during the entire processing period. Add more boiling water if needed to keep it at the required depth. As soon as processing time is up, remove the jars from the kettle. Set them a few inches apart on a thick towel or cooling rack. Do not set them in a draft or on a cool, wet surface. Once the jars are cool, wipe clean with a soapy cloth, and store until ready to use.

*Source: Home and Garden Bulletin No. 8 U.S. Department of Agriculture*

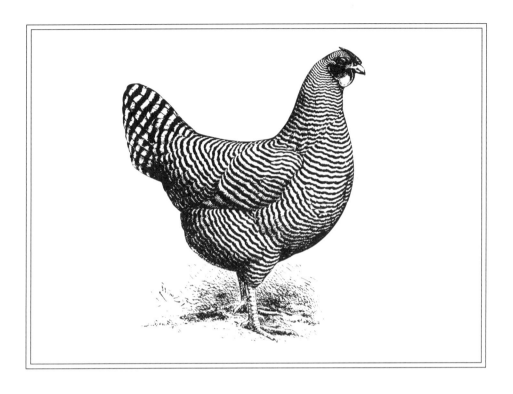

# POULTRY

# STRETCHING TO GET MOVING

First thing in the morning is a good time to stretch, loosen muscles, and better prepare yourself for a healthy day. Take a few minutes to stretch and you will feel better all day. Better yet, add about 15 minutes of aerobic exercise to your morning stretch routine. Swim, run, jump rope, or cycle 3 or 4 times a week to keep fit. Do not try to squeeze all your exercise into the weekend. If you cannot exercise every day, try every other day to improve overall fitness. You will feel better.

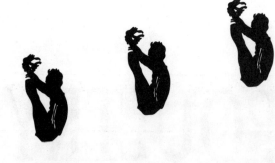

# DEFROSTING CHICKEN

The best method for defrosting a frozen chicken is the slowest. Leave chicken in its wrapper and let it thaw in the refrigerator; it will lose much less of its juice and flavor. If you are pressed for time, however, the best alternative is to unwrap it and thaw in a basin of cold running water. Remove the package of giblets from the cavity as soon as it can be pried loose.

## COOKING METHODS

| CHICKEN | USUAL WEIGHT | SUGGESTED COOKING METHODS |
|---|---|---|
| BROILER (2-3 months old) | 1½-2½ pounds | Broil, Grill, Roast |
| FRYER (3-5 months old) | 2-3 pounds | Fry, Roast, Sauté, Casserole, Poach |
| ROASTER (5½-9 months old) | Over 3 pounds | Roast, Poach, Fricassee |
| SQUAB CHICKEN or Baby Broiler (about 2 months old) | ¾-1 pound | Broil, Grill, Roast |
| STEWING CHICKEN (10-12 months old) | Usually over 3 pounds | Stew, Fricassee, Soup |

## ROASTING TIMETABLE

| UNDRESSED WEIGHT | SERVES | OVEN TEMP. | TIME |
|---|---|---|---|
| 1¼-2 lb. | 2 | 375° | 40-50 minutes |
| 2-3 lb. | 2-3 | 375° | 1-1½ hours |
| 3-4 lb. | 4 | 375° | 1-1¾ hours |
| 4½-6 lb. | 5-6 | 375° | 2-2¼ hours |

Stuffed chickens will need about 15 minutes longer.

## FREEZING

Buy the freshest birds and freeze them as soon as possible. Do not stuff a bird before freezing. Label and date, chickens will keep for 6 months at 0°F. or below. Commercially frozen chicken should be frozen in same wrappings until cooking time.

*Cooked Chicken* — Remove stuffing from chicken after cooking, cool both in refrigerator, then wrap them separately; use within a month.

# CURRY CHICKEN

4 servings

1 Tablespoon olive oil
$^1\!/_2$ cup onion — sliced
1 garlic clove — pressed
$^1\!/_2$ cup zucchini — unpeeled and sliced
$1^1\!/_2$ cups carrots — sliced thin
2 chicken breasts — remove skin and debone
1 cup potatoes — unpeeled and sliced
1 - $14^1\!/_2$ ounce can beef broth (or beef bouillon)
1 bay leaf
1-2 Tablespoons curry powder — depending on strength
$^1\!/_2$ cup raisins
1 Tablespoon fresh lemon juice
$^1\!/_2$ cup water
2 Tablespoons flour
$^1\!/_2$ cup apple — unpeeled and sliced

In a large saucepan, heat olive oil. Add onion, garlic, zucchini, and carrots. Cook 2-3 minutes. Cut chicken into chunks. Add chicken and potatoes to saucepan, and cook 2 minutes. Add beef broth, bay leaf, curry powder, raisins, and lemon juice. Mix water and flour together until smooth and add to mixture. Simmer about 10-15 minutes. Add apples and simmer about 15 minutes longer until vegetables are tender.

Great served alone or over rice or noodles.

Note: Try purchased beef broth without monosodium glutamate.

# CHICKEN STIR-FRY WITH BIFUN NOODLES

4 servings

2 Tablespoons olive oil or favorite unsaturated oil
2 large garlic cloves — minced
2-3 teaspoons fresh ginger root (depending on your taste for ginger)
    — peeled and chopped fine
2 whole chicken breasts — remove skin, debone, and cut in 1-inch
    chunks
¼ cup low-sodium soy sauce
3 tablespoons dried seaweed
1 cup cabbage — sliced thin
½ cup whole water chestnuts
½ cup bamboo shoots
½ cup white radish — cut into thin strips
1 package bifun noodles (Chinese-style noodles)

Heat oil in wok. Add garlic and ginger. Stir-fry for a few minutes.
Add chicken and soy sauce, cook for 3-5 minutes. Add seaweed,
cabbage, water chestnuts, bamboo shoots, and white radish. Continue to stir-fry until chicken is cooked thoroughly.
Meanwhile, bring a saucepan of water to a boil. Add package of
bifun noodles. Cook 2 minutes, remove from heat, and rinse with
cold water. Drain well and toss with stir-fry in wok. Heat
thoroughly. Serve hot.

# *SHIITAKE MARINATED CHICKEN*

2 servings

*2 chicken breasts — remove skin and debone*
*¹/₂ cup onion — sliced*
*1 bay leaf*
*5 thin slices of fresh ginger root*
*5 shiitake mushrooms (dried forest mushrooms) — soaked and*
  *sliced*
*1 Tablespoon brown sugar*
*1 garlic clove — pressed*
*¹/₂ cup white wine*
*1 cup water*

Preheat oven to 350°

Combine all ingredients in a large bowl, cover and marinate chicken 1-4 hours, depending on your schedule. Place chicken in baking dish, arrange mushrooms and onions on top of chicken. Pour marinade over chicken and bake for 45 minutes. Baste while cooking.

Note: Shiitake mushrooms can be found in Oriental section of supermarket, or in Asian stores.

# ROSEMARY CHICKEN

4 servings

1½-2 pounds of chicken breast, or assorted parts
1 can cream of mushroom soup
½ cup nonfat milk
½ cup onion — sliced
½ teaspoon dried rosemary — crushed
1 cup fresh mushrooms — washed and sliced
¼ teaspoon dried thyme
Pepper to taste

Preheat oven to 350°
Place chicken in a baking dish (remove skin to help lower fat). In a saucepan, heat cream of mushroom soup, milk, onion, rosemary, mushrooms, thyme, and pepper, mixing well. Pour mixture over chicken and cover with foil. Bake for 45 minutes.

# CHICKEN POTATO PIZZA

6 servings

*2 pounds chicken breasts — remove skin*
*2 Tablespoons fresh lemon juice*
*Pepper*
*3 cups raw potatoes — sliced*
*1 can cream of cheddar soup*
*½ cup nonfat milk*
*1 - 15 ounce can tomato sauce*
*1 teaspoon margarine*
*½ cup green onion — chopped*
*¼ teaspoon cayenne*
*¼ teaspoon ground cumin*
*½ teaspoon dried oregano*
*¼ cup green bell pepper — chopped*
*1 cup fresh mushrooms — sliced*
*¼ cup onion — chopped*
*½ cup skim mozzarella cheese — grated*
*½ cup lowfat swiss cheese — grated*

Preheat oven to 375°
Sprinkle chicken with lemon juice and pepper. Steam for 10 minutes, cool, remove chicken from bones, and cut into chunks. In the bottom of a 9x13 baking dish, place potatoes and chicken. In a saucepan, heat soup and milk, and pour over potatoes and chicken. In a saucepan, combine tomato sauce, margarine, green onion, cayenne, cumin, oregano, green bell pepper, mushrooms, and onions. Mix well. Simmer about 5 minutes. Pour over potatoes and chicken. Bake for 40 minutes. Top with cheeses and bake 15 minutes longer. Let stand 5 minutes after removing from oven before cutting and serving.

## TARRAGON GAME HENS

2 servings
(Whole hen per serving)

2 game hens
Pepper
1 Tablespoon fresh lemon juice
1½ cups carrots — quartered
1 cup broccoli florets
½ cup fresh orange juice
½ cup sherry
½ teaspoon dried tarragon

Preheat oven to 350°

Clean game hens, remove excess fat from inside and the skin from breasts; rinse. Place game hens in a baking dish, and sprinkle with pepper and lemon juice. Arrange carrots and broccoli around hens. In a small bowl, combine orange juice and sherry. Pour over hens and vegetables. Sprinkle with dried tarragon. Cover with foil and bake for 1½ hours. Baste occasionally.

## QUICK CHICKEN ENCHILADAS

4 servings

2 whole chicken breasts — remove skin and steam till done
2 fresh ears of corn (or 1 cup canned corn — drained)
½ cup black olives — sliced
⅓ cup onion — chopped
2 cans enchilada sauce (mild, medium, or hot)
1 package corn tortillas
¾ cup cheese — grated (use favorite lowfat cheese)

Preheat oven to 350°

Cool steamed chicken and cut into chunks. Cook fresh corn and remove corn from cob. In a bowl combine chicken, corn, olives, and onion. In a skillet, heat enchilada sauce; dip tortilla into sauce and remove. Add chicken filling, roll, place in baking dish, repeat until filling is used. Pour remaining enchilada sauce over tortillas, sprinkle with cheese. Bake until heated throughout, and cheese melts.

## CHICKEN STIR-FRY

4 servings

2 chicken breasts
1½ Tablespoons olive oil
¾ cup onion — sliced
¾ cup carrots — sliced thin
1½ cups yellow squash — sliced
1 Tablespoon fresh ginger root — chopped (use less if not familiar with ginger)
2-3 garlic cloves — chopped
¾ cup leeks — chopped
¾ cup celery — sliced
5 dried shiitake mushrooms — soaked for 20 minutes, drained and chopped
¼ cup low-sodium soy sauce
½ cup chicken broth

Skin and debone chicken breast and cut into chunks. In a skillet, heat oil, add chicken, onion, and carrots, and let sauté 2-3 minutes. Add remaining ingredients and simmer, covered, about 5 minutes, over medium heat. Serve with rice or pasta.

# BAKED MUSTARD CHICKEN WITH GARLIC CARROTS

4 servings

*1½-2 pounds whole chicken — remove most of skin*
*1½ Tablespoons dijon mustard*
*1½ Tablespoons spicy brown mustard*
*1 teaspoon prepared horseradish*
*2 tablespoons parmesan cheese — grated*
*1½ cups carrots — cut into serving-sized pieces*
*4 whole cloves of garlic — peeled*
*⅔ cup onion — chopped*
*¾ cup water*
*Pepper — optional*

Preheat oven to 350°

Rinse chicken. In a small bowl, combine dijon and brown mustards, horseradish, and cheese. Rub all over whole chicken. Place carrots over the bottom of a 9x13 baking dish, and add 4 whole garlic cloves. Place chicken on bed of carrots, sprinkle with onions. Add water to baking dish, sprinkle chicken with pepper if desired, cover and bake for 45 minutes. Remove cover and continue to cook for another 15 minutes.

# TURKEY BREAST WITH
# SPINACH STUFFING

4 servings

**STUFFING**

*1 Tablespoon olive oil*
*½ cup onion — chopped*
*1 Tablespoon green onion — chopped*
*2 Tablespoons leeks — chopped*
*4 slices of 7-grain bread (or whole wheat bread)*
*½ cup chicken broth*
*1 cup fresh spinach leaves — chopped*
*1 teaspoon dried sage*
*1 egg*
*Pepper*

*2 turkey breast halves — remove skin*
*1 cup carrots — cut into large pieces*
*½ cup onion — sliced*

Preheat oven to 350°

In a skillet, heat oil and sauté onion, green onion, and leeks until tender. In a bowl, crumble bread. Add onion sauté, chicken broth, spinach, sage, egg, and pepper to taste. Mix well. Divide in half. In a baking dish, place dressing in 2 mounds.

Place a turkey breast half over each mound of dressing, arrange carrots around turkey and place onion slices over top. Sprinkle with more pepper if desired. Cover with foil. Bake for ½ hour, remove foil, and continue baking for another ½ hour. Total cooking time: 1 hour. Test for doneness.

## QUICK BAKED CHICKEN

2 servings

*1 Tablespoon dijon mustard*
*1 Tablespoon safflower mayonnaise*
*2 chicken breasts — remove skin*
*2 cups fine bread crumbs*

Preheat oven to 350°

Mix mustard and mayonnaise in a bowl. Spread mixture over both sides of chicken breasts; dredge in bread crumbs. Place in a baking dish, cover with foil. Bake for 35-40 minutes. Remove foil for last 10 minutes of cooking time.

## ROLLED CHICKEN BREAST WITH FETTUCCINE

4 servings

**SAUCE** (make preferably in morning or day before)
*4-5 fresh tomatoes — chopped*
*$\frac{1}{4}$ cup red wine vinegar*
*Pinch of crushed red pepper*
*2 teaspoons fresh basil — chopped*
*$\frac{1}{2}$ teaspoon dried thyme*
*$\frac{1}{3}$ cup black olives — sliced*
*2 garlic cloves — chopped*
*$\frac{1}{3}$ cup raisins*

Combine all ingredients except raisins in a saucepan and simmer 1 hour over low heat. Add raisins and continue to simmer $\frac{1}{2}$ hour longer. (This is best if sauce sits overnight in refrigerator.)

## CHICKEN BREASTS

*1 cup onion — chopped*
*2 whole chicken breasts — remove skin and debone, cut in half (4)*
*3 garlic cloves — pressed*
*8 small broccoli florets — blanched*
*4 slices lowfat swiss cheese*

Preheat oven to 350°
Line a 9x13 baking dish with onions. Lay out half of chicken breast, rub each with garlic. Place two broccoli florets in center of each piece of chicken, and one-half piece of cheese at each end. Add 1 Tablespoon of sauce, and roll up each piece of chicken; place seam down on top of onions. Pour remaining sauce over chicken, cover with foil, and bake for 45 minutes. Remove foil and cook 5 minutes longer.

## FETTUCINE

*1/3 cup white wine*
*3 Tablespoons cream cheese*
*1/2 cup lowfat swiss cheese — shredded*
*Any reserved juice from baking chicken (above)*
*8-10 ounces pasta — cooked until tender, drained*
*Romano cheese — grated*

In a saucepan, heat white wine. Add cream cheese and mix until smooth. Add swiss cheese, and any sauce left in chicken baking dish. In a serving bowl, toss pasta with wine sauce, place baked chicken rolls on top, sprinkle with romano cheese and serve!

# BAKED CHICKEN WITH OYSTER SAUCE

2-3 servings

*½ cup oyster sauce*
*½ cup water*
*3 Tablespoons fresh lemon juice*
*1 teaspoon rosemary — chopped fine*
*1 teaspoon Pickapeppa sauce*
*3 garlic cloves — minced*
*2-2½ pounds chicken — cut into parts*
*2-2½ cups carrots — cut into sticks*
*½ cup onion — chopped*
*1 cup fresh white mushrooms — washed and quartered*

Preheat oven to 350°

In a bowl, combine oyster sauce, water, lemon juice, rosemary, Pickapeppa sauce, and garlic; mix well and set aside. Remove skin and excess fat from chicken, place chicken in oyster sauce mixture, and let sit 10 minutes or longer if time allows. Then place chicken parts in a 9x13 baking dish, arrange the carrots around the chicken, and arrange onions and mushrooms on top. Pour oyster sauce mixture over chicken, cover, and bake for 45-50 minutes, removing cover for last 5 minutes of cooking.

# TAMARIND CHICKEN

4 servings

*2 Tablespoons olive oil*
*½ teaspoon Worcestershire sauce*
*1 teaspoon low-sodium soy sauce*
*2 Tablespoons Tamarind fruit pulp — remove outer shell and seeds*
*2 pounds chicken breasts or whole chicken — cut up and remove*
  *skin*

352

*Pepper — optional*
*¹/₂ cup onion — sliced*
*¹/₂ cup fresh white mushrooms — washed and sliced*
*¹/₄ cup water*

Preheat oven to 350°

In a skillet, over medium heat, combine oil, Worcestershire sauce, soy sauce, and tamarind pulp. Let cook about a minute and add chicken pieces. Brown chicken on both sides and place in a baking dish. Add pepper, onions, and mushrooms to skillet, sauté a couple of minutes, and add ¹/₄ cup water, mixing well. Place onion mixture over chicken, cover, and bake for 45 minutes. Remove cover and cook 10 minutes longer. Terrific with rice.

---

# CHICKEN WITH GRAPES 
3-4 servings

*1 Tablespoon olive oil*
*4 garlic cloves — sliced*
*¹/₄ cup leeks — sliced*
*1¹/₂-2 pounds chicken breast — remove skin and debone*
*4 Tablespoons fresh lemon juice*
*1 Tablespoon sherry*
*1 Tablespoon tamari sauce (soy sauce)*
*2 Tablespoons raisins*
*³/₄-1 cup seedless grapes (green or purple) — washed and drained*

In a skillet, heat olive oil, garlic, and leeks. Let simmer about a minute. Cut chicken into 2-inch pieces. Add chicken, lemon juice, sherry, soy sauce, and raisins to skillet. Cover and let cook 4-5 minutes, or until chicken is done. Add grapes and cook a minute or so longer to warm grapes. Superb served with rice.

# PANCIT

1 Tablespoon olive oil
4 garlic cloves — diced
1 cup onion — sliced
½ cup chicken — parboiled and flaked
½ cup pork — parboiled and cut into thin strips
1½ Tablespoons low-sodium soy sauce
1 cup clam juice
2 Tablespoons fresh lemon juice
Pepper
1 cup cabbage — shredded
1 cup carrots — shredded
1 cup bean sprouts
1 cup celery — sliced
1 cup Chinese pea pods
1 package bifun noodles, or rice cake noodles, or ramen noodles
½ cup shrimp — rinsed and drained
1 lemon — for garnish

In a skillet, heat oil. Add garlic and onion, and sauté for 2 minutes. Add flaked chicken and strips of pork (set aside a small portion for garnish). Add soy sauce, clam juice, lemon juice, and pepper. Simmer 5 minutes. Add vegetables and simmer until almost done. Meanwhile, cook noodles, drain, place in hot skillet to dry, then remove and combine with chicken/pork mixture, mixing well. Add shrimp and cook until well heated. Arrange on platter and garnish with meat mixture previously set aside. Serve with lemon wedge as garnish.

# RAOUL'S CHICKEN FOR TWO

2 servings

*³/₄ cup fresh or canned pineapple — chopped*
*¹/₄ cup green onion — chopped*
*¹/₄ cup celery — chopped*
*10 thin slices fresh ginger root — pressed in garlic press*
*2 chicken breasts — remove skin*
*1 Tablespoon olive oil*
*2 Tablespoons low-sodium soy sauce*

Preheat oven to 350°

Cover the bottom of a baking dish with pineapple, green onion, celery, and half of ginger. Lay chicken on top. In a measuring cup, mix olive oil, soy sauce, and remaining ginger. Pour over top of chicken. Cover with foil and bake for 40 minutes.

# CHIN'S CHICKEN ORIENTAL

4 servings

*1¹/₂-2 pounds chicken — white or dark meat*
*¹/₂ cup oyster sauce*
*2 Tablespoons low-sodium soy sauce*
*4 drops sesame seed oil*
*¹/₂ cup white wine (or just plain water)*
*2 Tablespoons hoisin sauce*
*1 Tablespoon olive oil*
*Pepper — optional*

Remove chicken from bones and leave in large chunks. In a bowl, combine oyster sauce, soy sauce, sesame seed oil, white wine, and hoisin sauce. Mix well. Add chicken and marinate for 10 minutes. Remove chicken and place in skillet with heated oil, pour sauce over chicken and sprinkle with pepper. Cook about 20 minutes, uncovered, until chicken is done. Great served with rice.

# FAST BAKED CHICKEN

*Chicken — cut into parts*
*2-3 cloves garlic — pressed*
*1 Tablespoon olive oil*
*1 Tablespoon paprika*
*1-1¹/₂ teaspoons dried rosemary — crumbled*
*Pepper*

Preheat oven to 350°

This recipe is always good, and works for any size chicken. Remove the skin. Rub each piece of chicken with pressed garlic and olive oil. Mix paprika, rosemary, and pepper together. Rub mixture over each piece of chicken. Place in baking dish, cover, and bake for 35-40 minutes, or until chicken is well done.

---

## COLD CHICKEN STIR-FRY SALAD   4 servings

*1-1½ pounds chicken — white or dark meat*
*1 Tablespoon olive oil*
*4 drops sesame seed oil*
*½ cup onion — sliced*
*½ cup coconut milk*
*1-2 Tablespoons low-sodium soy sauce*
*Pepper*
*1 package bifun noodles — from Asian section of market*
*1 - 5 ounce can bamboo shoots — drained*
*1 - 5 ounce can water chestnuts — drained*
*¾ cup red bell pepper — cut into strips*
*1 cup snowpeas*

Remove chicken from bones and discard the skin. Cut chicken into large bite-sized pieces. Heat olive oil in skillet. Add sesame seed oil and onion. Sauté 1 minute. Add ¼ cup of coconut milk, chicken, soy sauce, and pepper. Simmer, uncovered, about 5 minutes. Meanwhile, cook bifun noodles in a pot of boiling water for about 2 minutes. Set aside to drain. Add to stir-fry: bamboo shoots, water chestnuts, bell pepper, snowpeas, and remaining ¼ cup coconut milk. Continue cooking 3-5 minutes longer. Add drained bifun noodles and toss well. Remove from heat and chill before serving.

# CHICKEN STRIPS

4 servings or 1 large salad

Excellent for salads, served over rice, or for finger food.

*5 dried forest mushrooms — shiitake*
*1½ cups flour*
*3 Tablespoons sesame seeds*
*½ teaspoon fresh ginger root — grated*
*Pepper*
*¼ cup low-sodium soy sauce*
*2 chicken breasts*
*4 Tablespoons leeks — chopped*
*1 Tablespoon olive oil*
*1 Tablespoon fresh lemon juice*

Soak dried mushrooms according to directions on package. In a bowl, mix flour, sesame seeds, ginger, and pepper. In another bowl, add soy sauce. Remove skin and bones from chicken. Cut into strips about 1 inch wide. Dip strips of chicken into soy sauce and then coat in flour mixture. In a skillet, heat olive oil; sauté leeks and sliced (soaked) mushrooms. Add chicken strips and drizzle with leftover soy sauce and lemon juice. Cook for 10 minutes.

# CHICKEN VERBIER

4-6 servings

*8-10 garlic cloves — diced*
*¹/₂ teaspoon paprika*
*¹/₂ teaspoon pepper*
*1 teaspoon olive oil*
*2 - 2 pound chickens — cut into parts*
*1 cup whole wheat or unbleached white flour*
*1 teaspoon olive oil — for browning*
*³/₄ cup onion — sliced thin*
*1 cup fresh mushrooms — sliced*
*1 tomato — chopped*
*4-5 Tablespoons parmesan cheese — grated*
*¹/₂ cup water*
*1 teaspoon dijon mustard*
*¹/₄ cup half-and-half*

Preheat oven to 350°

In a blender, combine garlic, paprika, pepper, and 1 teaspoon olive oil. Purée until smooth. Rub each piece of chicken with garlic purée. Dredge each piece of chicken in flour. In a skillet, heat 1 Tablespoon olive oil. Add chicken and brown on both sides. Place browned chicken in a baking dish, and cover with sliced onions, mushrooms, and chopped tomato; sprinkle with cheese. Add water to baking dish, cover with foil, and bake for 45 minutes. Remove foil and let bake 15 minutes longer. Check chicken for doneness. Place chicken on a platter and cover to keep warm. Pour drippings from baking dish into a skillet. Add mustard and half-and-half, mix well and simmer 3-4 minutes to thicken. Pour thickened sauce over chicken on platter and serve.

Great with rice, potatoes, or pasta.

# ROASTED CHICKEN WITH BRUSSELS SPROUTS

4 servings

1<sup>1</sup>/<sub>2</sub>-2 *pounds whole chicken*
<sup>1</sup>/<sub>2</sub> *teaspoon dried thyme*
*Pepper to taste*
<sup>1</sup>/<sub>2</sub> *cup water*
<sup>1</sup>/<sub>2</sub> *cup onion — sliced*
1<sup>1</sup>/<sub>2</sub>-2 *cups Brussels sprouts — wash and remove damaged leaves,*
    *trim bottoms, if large cut in half*
1 *Tablespoon honey*

Preheat oven to 350°

Remove excess fat and skin from chicken. Rinse and pat dry. Sprinkle with thyme and pepper. Place chicken in a baking dish. Add water to baking dish and top chicken with onions. Cover with foil and let bake about 25 minutes. Add Brussels sprouts around chicken in baking dish. Drizzle honey over chicken, cover and continue to bake 20-25 minutes longer.

# MARINADE FOR CHICKEN, SEAFOOD OR BEEF

*⅓ cup sherry*
*¼ cup low-sodium soy sauce*
*½ cup water*
*2 Tablespoons fresh ginger root — peeled and grated*
*3 Tablespoons orange juice*
*2 Tablespoons green onion — chopped*
*2 Tablespoons brown sugar*

Marinate at least 1 hour, then either bake, barbecue or fry.

# JEANNIE'S CHICKEN OR STEAK SPRAY

*1 cup sweet vermouth*
*2 Tablespoons Worcestershire sauce*
*2 Tablespoons low-sodium soy sauce*
*½ teaspoon liquid smoke*

Combine all ingredients. Spray chicken or steak while cooking, turning often.
For variations, try substituting apricot brandy or vodka for the sweet vermouth.

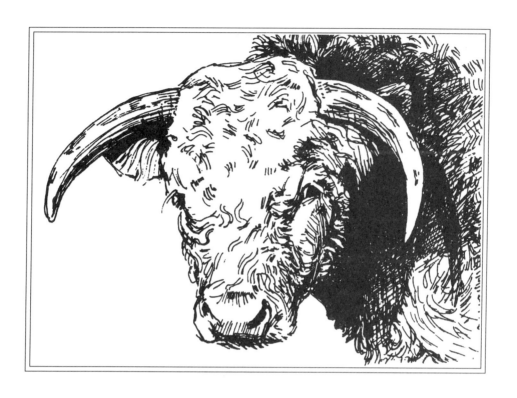

# MEAT

# CROSS COUNTRY SKIING

Cross country skiing is the best aerobic sport around. It puts arms and legs, abdominal muscles, and almost every part of the body through an intensive workout.

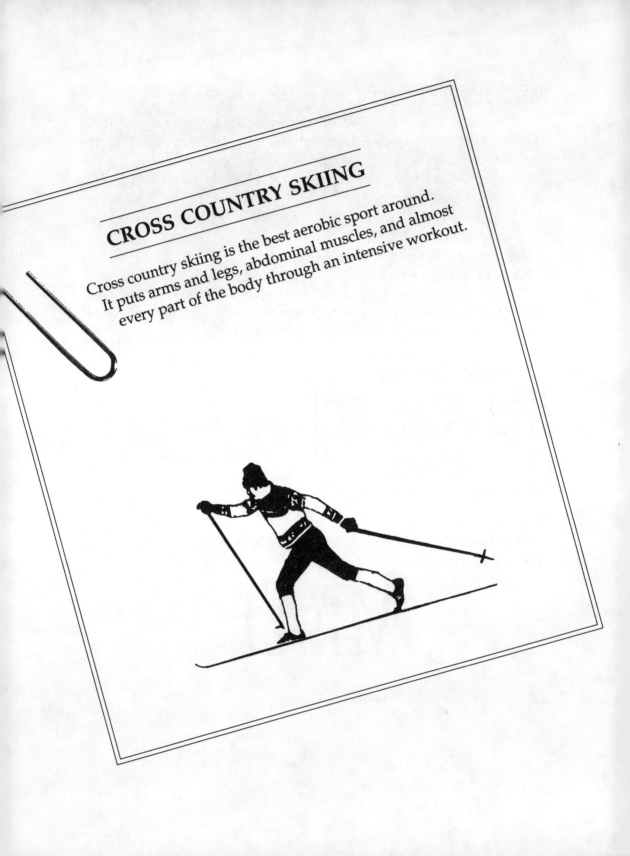

## MEAT SELECTION

Fat is one of the most critical elements determining meat grade. The reason some carcasses are rated lower is, ironically, that they are lower in fat content. High fat content, evenly dispersed through the carcass (good marbling), gives a cut of meat more tenderness, flavor, juiciness, and, of course, more cholesterol.

The benefit of buying lower grade meats for the fat-conscious consumer is twofold.

- Better nutritionally, lower in fat.
- Lower in price than the "top-of-the-line" grades.

A voluntary program called the Uniform Retail Meat Industry Standards helps shoppers identify cuts of meat through encouraging standard labeling at supermarkets.

```
┌──────────────────────────────────────┐
│                                        │
│        MEAT DEPARTMENT                 │
│                                        │
│   Weight        ── PAY ──       PRICE  │
│   Lb Net                        Per Lb │
│                ┌─────────┐             │
│   0.00         │ $0.00   │     0.00    │
│                └─────────┘             │
│          BEEF CHUCK                    │
│          BLADE ROAST                   │
│                                        │
└──────────────────────────────────────┘
```

The first word or words on the meat label will indicate the kind of meat — beef, pork, lamb, or veal.

The next information indicates the primal cut, which is the cut made at the slaughter house.

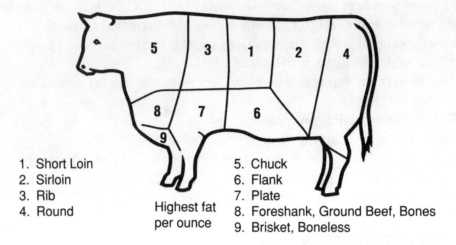

1. Short Loin
2. Sirloin
3. Rib
4. Round

Highest fat
per ounce

5. Chuck
6. Flank
7. Plate
8. Foreshank, Ground Beef, Bones
9. Brisket, Boneless

The last line of the label indicates the retail cut (the cut made by the grocery store) — blade roast, spare ribs, loin chops, for example.

Tougher meats with lower fat content require longer, moister cooking to tenderize them, although they have just as many vitamins and minerals as the most tender T-bone. Try stewing, simmering, or poaching these meats. Marinating or pounding the meat will help tenderize it, and slicing thinly across the grain when serving will also improve the taste.

**LOWEST FAT CUTS**
*Beef* — Top Round, Flank, Top Sirloin, Tip, Extra Lean Ground
*Pork* — Tenderloin, Loin Chops, Leg (Fresh Ham)
We, as consumers concerned about fat intake, can take protective measures to have our meat and enjoy it too, by:
• Buying lowfat cuts
• Trimming excess fat before cooking
• Choosing broiling over frying

*Source: American Institute for Cancer Research, Newsletter, Winter 1986, Issue 14.*

# SLOW-COOKED LAMB ROAST

4 servings

*2-3 pound lamb roast*
*2-3 garlic cloves — crushed*
*2 Tablespoons dried rosemary — crushed*
*1 Tablespoon coarsely ground pepper*
*³/₄ cup parmesan cheese, grated*
*1 cup onion — chopped*
*¹/₂ cup water*

Preheat oven to 300°

Rub pressed garlic (use pulp) over all sides of roast. Mix rosemary and pepper together and rub on all sides of roast; then place roast in a baking dish. Pat cheese thickly on top and sides of roast. Place onions around and on top of roast. Add water to baking dish and cover with foil. Bake for 3 hours.

Note: This is a great recipe to pop into the oven and let cook while doing errands. When short on time, raise temperature and cut time down accordingly.

# CURRIED LAMB STEW

4 servings

1 Tablespoon olive oil
1 pound lamb stew meat — trimmed of excess fat and cut into large
    pieces
1 large garlic clove — pressed
½ cup onion — chopped
¾ cup carrots — sliced
½ cup apple — sliced
1½ cups small raw potatoes — sliced
1 bunch of fresh asparagus spears — chopped into large pieces
    (8-12 spears)
2 Tablespoons whole wheat flour
1 cup water
½ cup raisins
Pepper
1 Tablespoon curry powder — if not familiar with curry powder,
    use less and keep tasting

In a large saucepan, heat oil. Add lamb, garlic, and onion. Brown meat slightly. Add carrots, apple, potatoes, and asparagus. Blend 2 Tablespoons flour with 1 cup of water until smooth. Add to saucepan and stir. Add raisins, pepper, and curry powder. Simmer 25-35 minutes, or until lamb is tender. Use more water if needed for desired consistency.

Note: Beef may be used instead of lamb.

# BROILED LAMB STEAKS

4-6 servings
(depending on size)

*4-6 lamb steaks*
*1 teaspoon fresh lemon juice*
*½ teaspoon dried tarragon*
*¼ teaspoon dried mint*
*¼ teaspoon coarsely ground pepper*

Arrange steaks on broiler pan and sprinkle with lemon juice. In a small dish, mix together tarragon, mint, and pepper, and sprinkle over tops of steaks. Place about 4 inches from broiler. Broil 2-3 minutes on each side.

## ZUCCHINI-CARROT MEAT LOAF     4 servings

3 teaspoons tomato paste
3/4 cup water
1 teaspoon dried thyme
1/4 teaspoon dried rosemary — crushed
Pepper to taste
1/2 cup lowfat swiss cheese — grated
1/2 cup carrots — grated
1/2 cup zucchini — grated
1/2 cup bran
1 pound lean ground beef
1 egg
1 teaspoon Worcestershire sauce

Preheat oven to 350°

In a bowl, mix tomato paste with water. Add thyme, rosemary, pepper, cheese, carrots, zucchini, bran, ground beef, egg, and Worcestershire sauce. Mix well. Shape into desired loaf or place in loaf pan and bake for 1 hour and 10 minutes. Cool at least 5 minutes before slicing.

## ASPARAGUS AND SPINACH MEAT LOAF     4 servings

1 cup fresh spinach
1 pound lean ground beef
1 egg
3-5 fresh mushrooms — sliced
4 asparagus spears — raw and chopped
1/4 cup bran

¼ *cup black olives — sliced*
**Pepper to taste**
½ *teaspoon dried rosemary — crushed*
½ *teaspoon lemon juice — fresh*

Preheat oven to 350°

Blanch spinach in boiling water for 1 minute. Squeeze out excess water, then chop. Mix spinach, beef, egg, mushrooms, asparagus, bran, olives, pepper, rosemary, and lemon juice. Mix well, shape into loaf or place in loaf pan, and bake for 45 minutes-1 hour. Cool 5 minutes before slicing.

---

# RAY'S PEPPER STEAK 4-5 servings

½ *cup unbleached white or whole wheat flour*
½ *teaspoon salt (optional)*
*1 teaspoon pepper*
*2-3 pounds round steak (or desired cut)*
*1 Tablespoon olive oil*
*2 garlic cloves — chopped*
*1 cup water*
*1 Tablespoon Worcestershire sauce*
*1 cup onion — diced*
*2 cups green bell pepper — cut into strips*

In a bowl, mix flour, salt, and pepper. Cut steak into strips and dredge in flour mixture. In a skillet, heat oil. Add steak and garlic, and brown. Add water and simmer on medium-low until meat is tender. Add Worcestershire sauce, onion, and green pepper. Simmer until bell peppers are tender.
Great served over rice.

# HERB SPAGHETTI MEAT SAUCE

6 servings

1 Tablespoon olive oil
1/2 cup onion — chopped
2 Tablespoons garlic — chopped
1/4 cup leek — chopped
1/4 cup fresh chives — chopped
2 Tablespoons fresh basil — chopped (or 1 Tablespoon dried)
1 teaspoon dried green oregano
1 Tablespoon dried thyme
2 - 8 ounce cans salt-free tomato sauce
1 - 16 ounce can salt-free tomatoes
1/3 cup sherry
2/3 cup water
1 cup green pepper — chopped
1 cup fresh mushrooms — chopped
1 pound lean ground beef

In a large saucepan, heat oil. Add onion, garlic, leek, chives, basil, oregano, and thyme. Sauté until onions are clear and tender. Add tomato sauce, tomatoes, sherry, water, green pepper, and mushrooms. Simmer over medium heat. Meanwhile lightly brown the beef and stir into sauce mixture. Simmer for 45 minutes.

# SLOPPY JOES

*1¹/₂-2 pounds lean ground beef*
*¹/₂ cup leeks — chopped*
*1 cup onion — chopped*
*2 garlic cloves — pressed, use pulp*
*2 cups celery — diced*
*¹/₂ cup chili sauce*
*¹/₂ cup ketchup*
*1³/₄ cups water*
*2 Tablespoons Worcestershire sauce*
*2 Tablespoons red wine vinegar — optional*
*1 Tablespoon brown sugar*
*2 teaspoons dry mustard*
*1 teaspoon paprika*
*1 Tablespoon chili powder*
*2 teaspoons fresh parsley — chopped*
*Pepper — to taste*
*1 teaspoon fresh lemon juice*

In a skillet, brown ground beef with leeks, onion, and garlic. Add rest of ingredients and simmer about 1 hour. Serve on buns.

# MEATBALLS (HIGH FIBER)

4 servings

1 pound lean ground beef
$1/2$ cup onion — chopped
3 garlic cloves — diced
$1/4$ cup green bell pepper — chopped
Pepper
1 teaspoon dried thyme
$1/8$ cup wheat germ
$1/8$ cup bran
$1/4$ cup oats
1 egg
$1/2$ cup whole wheat flour

In a bowl, combine ground beef, onion, garlic, green pepper, pepper, thyme, wheat germ, bran, oats, and egg.
Form meatballs (about 1 Tablespoon each of mixture), and dredge in flour. In a skillet, heat olive oil and brown meatballs on all sides. Cook until well done. Serve as is or with your favorite sauce.

# SAUTÉED VENISON

4 servings

*1½ pounds deer meat*
*¼ cup whole wheat flour*
*¼ cup unbleached white flour*
*½ teaspoon garlic powder*
*½ teaspoon coarsely ground pepper*
*2 Tablespoons olive oil*

Cut venison into desired size pieces. In a bowl, combine flours, garlic powder, and pepper. Dredge deer meat pieces in flour and place on a platter. Let sit in refrigerator for 1 hour before frying. In a skillet, heat oil, add deer meat and cook until done, browning on both sides.

## STORAGE OF GAME

To prolong the delights of the hunt, store the surplus to prevent waste. Frozen storage is the best method. Preservation of the flavor and texture of a frozen product will depend on how well it is wrapped and sealed, where you store it, temperature, and, of course, length of storage.

Game is cut and cleaned by the same methods as domestic meats, and requires the same treatment as beef. When the carcass is thoroughly chilled, cut into family-sized portions. Wash, chill, and wrap in moisture- and vapor-proof paper, or aluminum foil. Ordinary wrapping paper or waxed paper will not do.

# INDEX

**378**

**381**

Please send "Whole Foods Kitchen Journal"

_____ copies at $ **18.95**___ each = _____

Shipping = _____

Washington residents
add 8% sales tax = _____

Total = _____

Mail your orders to:  Elfin Cove Press
P.O. Box 924
Redmond, Washington 98073-0924

Ship ordered books to (please print):

Name_____

Address_____

City_____State_____Zip_____

Please make payment by check or money order. We also accept
MasterCard and Visa.

Visa / MasterCard (circle one)

Card Number_____ Exp. Date_____

Signature_____

❑ Gift card enclosed.